KETO DIET FOR BEGINNERS

A Unique Collection of More than 100 Delicious Keto Diet Recipes For Rapid Weight Loss

WAYNE A. COLE

ISBN - 9798671065275

TABLE OF CONTENTS

Introduction..7

What is the Keto Diet?...8

How Does the Keto Diet Work?.....................................9

Fat Burning Mode...9

Entering Ketosis...9

What Are the Advantages of a Keto Diet?....................11

Who is This Diet For?..13

Top Tips for Keto Success...14

Breakfast...15

    Cheesy Scrambled Eggs:...16

    Keto Coconut Porridge:...17

    Eggs Benedict on Sliced Avocado:............................18

    Cauliflower Hash Browns:...19

    Banana Waffles:...20

    Eggy Breakfast Muffins:..21

    Chia Seed Pudding:...22

    Nutty Granola:...23

    No-Nuts Keto Bread:...24

Keto French Toast...25

    Mug Bread:..26

    French Toast Batter:..27

    Mexican Breakfast Eggs:...28

    Bacon and Egg Breakfast Cups:................................29

    Boiled Eggs with Asparagus Dippers:.......................30

    Classic Bacon and Eggs:...31

Smoothies and Breakfast Drinks....................................32

    Spiced Pumpkin Latte:..33

    Homemade Electrolyte Lemonade:...........................33

Super-Greens Breakfast Smoothie: 34

Flavoured Water: 34

Thirst Quenching Ice Tea: 35

Classic Coffee with Cream: 35

Keto Friendly Hot Chocolate: 36

Blueberry Breakfast Smoothie: 36

Vanilla Ice latte 37

Strawberry Milkshake: 37

Lunch 38

Cheesy Croque Madame: 39

Mushroom and Bacon Slice: 40

Crispy Kale and Bacon Bowl with a Fried Egg: 41

Spinach Frittata: 42

Cloud Bread: 43

Bacon, Lettuce and Tomato Sandwiches (with Cloud Bread): 44

Cheese and Red Onion Sandwich with Cloud Bread: 44

No Bake Salmon and Avocado Boats: 45

Tuna Plate: 46

Baked Goats Cheese Salad: 47

Prawn Deviled Eggs: 48

Caesar Salad: 49

Creamy Cauliflower Salad: 50

Crunchy Walnut and Courgette Salad: 51

Traditional Nicoise Salad: 52

Baked Salmon with Creamy Pesto Dressing: 53

Tomato and Parmasan Soup: 54

Winter Warmer Chicken Soup: 55

Creamy Broccoli and Leek Soup: 56

Chicken Wings with Chipotle Aioli: 57

Dinner 58

Pan Fried Chicken Breast with Herb Butter: 59

Pork, Onion and Green Pepper Stir Fry: 60

Indian Chicken Korma Curry: 61

Pork Sausages with Creamy Cabbage Mash: 62

Broccoli and Cauliflower Cheese with Sausage:....................................63
Keto Lasagna:....................................64
Scallops With Herb Butter:....................................65
Spicy Prawn Salad:....................................66
Brussel Sprouts with Bacon and Red Onion:....................................67
Baked Brie with Walnuts and Rosemary:....................................68
Turnip Gratin:....................................69
Pork Chops with Buttery Green Beans:....................................70
Chicken and Broccoli Stir Fry:....................................70
Roast Chicken with Garlic and Herb Butter:....................................71
Mexican Chilli Stuffed Peppers with Cheese:....................................72

Sauces, Dips and Condiments 73
Easy Keto Bechamel Sauce:....................................74
Low- Carb Tomato Sauce:....................................75
Infused Olive Oil:....................................76
Homemade Almond-Butter:....................................77
Avocado Hummus:....................................78
Alfredo Sauce:....................................79
Hollandaise Sauce:....................................80
Caesar Salad Dressing:....................................81
Herb Butter:....................................81
Nicoise Salad Dressing:....................................82
Creamy Mustard Vinaigrette 82
Very Versatile Creamy Salad Dressing 83
Chipotle Aioli:....................................83
Keto Friendly Raspberry Jam:....................................84
Eggplant Dip:....................................85

Desserts....................................86
Dark Chocolate Cups:....................................87
Fresh Berries with Whipped Cream:....................................87
Chocolate Macadamia BonBons:....................................88
Spiced Chai Truffle Balls:....................................89
Lemon Ice Cream:....................................90
Vanilla Bean Panna Cotta:....................................90

Blueberry Ice Cream: 91

Cinnamon Apple Trifle: 92

Avocado Chocolate Truffles: 93

Summer Berry Crumble Pots: 94

Chocolate Fudge Bars: 95

Fruity Frozen Yoghurt: 96

Griddled Hot Peaches with Cream: 96

Nutty Granola Bars with Dark Chocolate: 97

Chocolate and Raspberry Mousse: 98

Snacks 99

Cheese Crisps: 100

Halloumi and Bacon Bites: 100

Garlic Bread 101

Vegetable Sticks with Avocado Hummus: 101

Spicy Roast Nuts 102

Homemade Pork Scratchings: 102

Spicy Courgette Crisps: 103

Mug Bread Cracker Thins with Dip: 103

Kale Chips: 104

Seeded Parmesan Chips: 104

Grilled Cheese Sandwich 105

Chia Seed Pudding with Fresh Berries: 105

No-Nuts Toast with Butter: 106

Boiled Eggs with Mayonnaise: 106

Salad Wrap Bites: 107

Disclaimer 108

INTRODUCTION

It can be so difficult finding a successful diet plan that fits into our busy modern lifestyle, but search no more as the ketogenic diet could be the answer to your prayers! This simple, no nonsense diet is based around scientific facts and delicious, homemade meals made with tasty ingredients.

Gone are the days of microwave dinners, meal replacement shakes and exhausting gym routines. This keto Diet really could change your life as it has done for millions of others around the world already!

Read on to find out a little bit more about how the keto diet works and who it's suitable for! We've already done all the hard work for you, by compiling over 100 delicious keto-friendly recipes for you to try out! We've got breakfast, lunch, and dinner sorted, as well as recipes for keto-friendly sauces, dips, smoothies and refreshing drinks.

So, what are you waiting for? Start the keto diet today!

WHAT IS THE KETO DIET?

Unlike many modern diet plans, the main principles of the keto Diet are simple. The emphasis is on maintaining a high-fat, low-carb diet.

In many ways, it's similar to other low-carb diets, past and present! Remember the Atkins Diet? It's like the modernised version of that well known classic. However, we now have the science behind how this diet actually works, and the findings are fascinating.

We start by:

- Eating substantially fewer carbohydrates
- Maintaining medium or average protein intake
- Dramatically increasing 'good' fat consumption

HOW DOES THE KETO DIET WORK?

A sudden and notable reduction in carbohydrates will essentially kick start your body into a metabolic state called 'ketosis'. When your body is in a state of ketosis, it uses fat as opposed to sugar (glucose) as its main source of fuel or energy.

Fat Burning Mode

Essentially what you're doing is starving your body of its usual energy source, which is glucose (comes from sugar and carbohydrates). Your body is forced to look for other sources of energy, so it turns to fat. The fat stored in your body, together with the fat consumed in your diet, is suddenly burned for energy instead of carbohydrates. This is the reason that ketosis is often referred to as your body's "fat-burning mode", aiding fast and efficient weight loss, even without hitting the gym.

When we eat carbohydrates, the glucose from our food either gets used straight away, or it gets stored in the liver and gradually released when needed for energy. This has worked beautifully for many years, but our diets have changed a lot over the last few decades. These days we have an abundance of processed carbs and high-sugar foods and drinks at our disposal, which are some of the main causes for weight-gain, as well as many other health problems.

Entering Ketosis

After we've ditched the carbs, the glucose stores in the liver become depleted. Our body can't enter the state of ketosis until the glucose stores have been used up. On average, it takes people around three days to enter ketosis. We'll be honest with you at this point and tell you that many people struggle getting past day three because of something we call the "keto flu".

As your body runs out of glucose and before it switches into fat burning mode, it's not uncommon for us to feel lethargic and even a bit cranky. Thankfully, there are ways in which we can avoid these keto flu symptoms, before ketosis comes to the rescue, sourcing energy from fat instead. For more information on avoiding the keto flu, see our top tips for keto success.

Our liver produces low amounts of ketone enzymes all the time, as a way of keeping us going when our glucose levels are low, like when we're asleep, intermittent fasting, or even if we've just skipped a meal when we are busy!

The ketones only do the job for as long as they are needed and as soon as we begin to eat carbohydrates again, the body switches back to running on glucose as its main 'fuel source'.

After dramatically reducing carbohydrate intake for a certain amount of time (usually three to four days), we can enter the true nutritional ketosis metabolic state. When you're in ketosis, your liver is producing enough ketones to happily fuel your body throughout the day!

Once your body has fully switched to ketosis, you will find that you have bundles more energy than you used to have, Not only that, but you'll no longer experience the highs and lows that come with eating carbs. No more sugar crashes and no more sleepy afternoons in the office after lunch as ketones are a much more stable and consistent energy source.

You can also wave goodbye to the 'hangry' feeling you get when you've not eaten in a few hours! Many people notice that they feel less hungry on a ketogenic diet, and subsequently, snack a lot less!

WHAT ARE THE ADVANTAGES OF A KETO DIET?

The advantages of a ketogenic diet should already be becoming more clear.

Some of the established benefits are:

- **Rapid weight loss:** Once in a ketogenic state, the body shifts to burning fat as its main fuel source! Your body will literally start using your unwanted fat for energy! Paired this with your reduced appetite (see below), many people notice the weight just melting off in a matter of weeks, without counting calories, a fancy exercise regime, or going hungry!

- **A more regulated and reduced appetite:** Although initially entering the 'ketogenic state' can be frustrating (keto flu, cravings and irritability are common side effects of low glucose). Once there, one of the first things people notice is that they are no longer anywhere near as hungry as they used to feel. It is now proven in trials that being in ketosis substantially suppresses our appetite. It's so much easier to lose weight when we're not having cravings all the time!

- **An improvement, or even reversal of type two diabetes and pre-diabetes:** It has been proven that diabetic patients following a strict low-carb diet can help 'normalise' their insulin response and blood sugar levels, potentially reversing the damage caused by pre-diabetes, or leading to no longer having to take daily medication!

- **Simple to follow:** When you first start the keto diet, you will need to spend a bit of time getting to know the foods that are keto-friendly and the foods that aren't. We all know that bread, pasta, and potatoes are high carb foods, but did you know that mangos, bananas, and raisins were super high carb too? It's easy to learn which foods to avoid though and many people much prefer the foods available on this diet as opposed to others (think bacon, eggs, steak, cheese… Yum!). Also, with the help of this book, you'll never be stuck for meal inspiration and recipes again!

- **Inexpensive:** Another advantage to the keto diet is that it isn't expensive to follow, especially compared to diets that require you to buy special meals and shakes!

WAYNE A. COLE

WHO IS THIS DIET FOR?

We believe the keto diet it's for just about everyone! Many people are recommended a low carb diets for health reasons, but the most common reason for people choosing keto above all others is for dramatic and fast weight loss.

There have been some amazing health claims over the years, and research suggests just a few weeks of a strict ketogenic diet can improve symptoms of type 2 diabetes, pre-diabetes, migraine headaches, hormonal imbalances causing PCOS in women, assist in seizure management for those with epilepsy and possibly even slowing down the effects of Alzheimers!

And as we mentioned before, it's an easy diet to follow! It's convenient, simple, and best of all, it allows you to eat many foods that would be banned on other diets!

So, why not give it a go? What do you have to lose?

TOP TIPS FOR KETO SUCCESS

Try and reduce your daily 'net-carb' intake: Studies have proven that eating fewer than 20 grams of net carbs every day can assist in achieving 'nutritional ketosis' in around 2-3 days. The sooner you kick the carbs and enter ketosis, the happier you'll be! All nutritional information can be found alongside our handy recipes in this book.

Don't be scared of fat: Eating a substantial amount of fat is an important part of the ketogenic diet! If you're worried about 'bad' fats, you can try and stick to healthier plant-based fats such as olive oil, nuts, avocado and coconut milk!

Have a go at intermittent fasting: Try having a go at intermittent fasting at the beginning of your diet as this can kick start the ketosis transition. Fasting for 12-15 hours without eating can seem daunting, but you only need to do it at the beginning to ensure a quick and easy switch from glucose to ketones. It can be as easy as skipping breakfast or having an early dinner!

Avoid the keto flu: Staying hydrated is absolutely key in avoiding keto flu symptoms! The low carb nature of this diet leads to increased water loss and decreased water retention, so you need to make sure you stock up on electrolytes and drink plenty of water. Eat nutrient dense foods, plenty of fat and calories, and exercise gently. You may also find that sleeping more helps in those first few days of ketosis, as your body gets used to its new energy source.

So, what are you waiting for? The world of keto awaits you. We hope this handy recipe book will inspire your new found love of cooking carb-free!

BREAKFAST

CHEESY SCRAMBLED EGGS:

PREP TIME: 3 MIN / COOKING TIME: 5 MIN / SERVINGS: 2 / SERVING SIZE: 1 CUP
CALORIES: 400 / NET CARBS: 2G / FIBRE: 0G / FAT: 40G / PROTEIN: 15G

Recipe Note: *These eggs are incredibly simple but come out perfect every time! Try adding smoked salmon, sauteed mushrooms or a few buttery pan fried cherry tomatoes if you want to take this recipe to the next level!*

INGREDIENTS:

- 50g // 2oz salted butter
- 4 eggs
- 15g // 0.5oz cheddar cheese
- chopped fresh herbs, such as chives or parsley
- pinch of sea salt and pepper

METHOD:

1. Crack eggs into a bowl and whisk with a fork until frothy and combined.

2. In a non-stick frying pan, melt the butter on a low heat. Once fully melted pour in the egg mixture and sprinkle on the cheese.

3. After about 30 seconds use a spatula to gently fold and stir the eggs, letting the cheese melt.

4. When the eggs look like they're almost finished, take them off the heat and set aside. The trick is to take the eggs off a little early, as they continue to cook in the warm pan.

5. Serve eggs on a plate, garnish with chopped fresh herbs and salt and pepper to taste.

WAYNE A. COLE

KETO COCONUT PORRIDGE:

PREP TIME: 5 MIN / COOKING TIME: 5 MIN / SERVINGS: 1 / SERVING SIZE: 1 CUP
CALORIES: 642 / NET CARBS: 4G / FIBRE: 5G / FAT: 64G / PROTEIN: 12G

INGREDIENTS:

- 12g // 1tbsp chia seeds
- 10g // 1tbsp sesame seeds
- 1 egg
- 75ml // ⅓ cup coconut cream
- 30g // 1oz coconut oil
- Pinch of salt

METHOD:

1. Mix all of your weighed out ingredients, apart from the coconut oil, in a bowl. Whisk with a fork to break up the egg. Let it sit for 5 minutes for the chia seeds to absorb some of the moisture.

2. Add the coconut oil to a small saucepan and let it melt gently.

3. Pour in the wet ingredients and gently sir until thickening up and simmering. Don't let it boil!

4. Serve with a sprinkle of toasted coconut flakes, cinnamon or a dollop of our keto-friendly raspberry jam!

EGGS BENEDICT ON SLICED AVOCADO:

PREP TIME: 10 MIN / COOKING TIME: 5 MIN / SERVINGS: 4 / SERVING SIZE: 1
CALORIES: 522 / NET CARBS: 3G / FIBRE: 7G / FAT: 48G / PROTEIN: 16G

Recipe Note: *Hollandaise Sauce isn't just for eggs benedict! You can use it as a delicious sauce to accompany fish, chicken and steak dinners too!*

Vegetarians can swap out the smoked salmon and replace it with wilted spinach for the 'Eggs Florentine' version of this dish! You can also experiment with adding ham or bacon for a more traditional eggs benedict.

INGREDIENTS:

- 2 ripe avocados
- 4 eggs
- 1 tbsp white vinegar
- 150g // 5oz smoked salmon
- 4 tbsp Hollandaise Sauce

METHOD:

1. Bring a pot of water to the boil. Once it's bubbling nicely, turn the temperature down and let simmer. Add the white vinegar to the water.

2. Crack 1 egg at a time into a large spoon or shallow cup. This makes it easier to gently tip the egg into the boiling water without breaking the yolk. Add each egg gently to the water and poach for 2-3 minutes for a runny yolk or 4-5 minutes for a hard yolk.

3. Remove the eggs with a slotted spoon and place on a piece of kitchen paper to dry and absorb some of the water.

4. Cut the avocados in half and remove the pits. Slice thinly and arrange on each plate.

5. Top with an egg, a few slices of smoked salmon and a generous dollop of home made hollandaise sauce! You can sprinkle with extra seasoning and some chopped fresh herbs!

CAULIFLOWER HASH BROWNS:

PREP TIME: 10 MIN / COOKING TIME: 30 MIN / SERVINGS: 4 / SERVING SIZE: 1-2
CALORIES: 282 / NET CARBS: 5G / FIBRE: 3G / FAT: 26G / PROTEIN:7G

INGREDIENTS:

- 450g // 1lb cauliflower
- 3 eggs
- ½ yellow onion, sliced finely
- 110g // 4oz salted butter
- Salt and pepper

METHOD:

1. Wash and trim the leaves and stalk from the cauliflower. Coarsely grate the cauliflower head into a bowl.

2. Add the remaining ingredients and mix well. Set aside for 5-10 minutes.

3. In a large flat base frying pan, add a generous amount of butter and heat on the stove. Once the butter is melted and bubbling, spoon dollops of the cauliflower mixture into the pan and flatten into neat little 3-4 inch diameter circles.

4. Fry for 5 minutes on each side until crispy and golden! Don't try and move or flip the hash browns too quickly or they may fall apart!

5. Serve with chopped herbs and a dollop of sour cream. These hash browns are also great with bacon and eggs in a keto-friendly english breakfast!

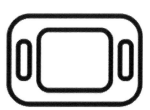

BANANA WAFFLES:

PREP TIME: 10 MIN / COOKING TIME: 20 MIN / SERVINGS: 8 / SERVING SIZE: 1-2
CALORIES: 155 / NET CARBS: 4G / FIBRE: 2G / FAT: 13G / PROTEIN: 5G

INGREDIENTS:

- 1 ripe banana
- 4 eggs
- 100g // ¾ cup almond flour
- 175ml // ¾ cup coconut milk
- 5g // 1tsp baking powder
- 1 pinch of salt
- ½ tsp vanilla essence
- 1tsp ground cinnamon
- Coconut oil for frying

METHOD:

1. Add all ingredients to a big bowl and beat together until they form a smooth creamy batter.

2. You can use a traditional waffle iron, or a frying pan if you don't have one! Add a little coconut oil and fry until the waffles are golden brown and cooked all the way through.

3. You can serve them with a dollop of whipped coconut cream and fresh berries, or why not try with our home-made almond butter or sugar-free raspberry jam.

EGGY BREAKFAST MUFFINS:

PREP TIME: 5 MIN / COOKING TIME: 20 MIN / SERVINGS: 6 / SERVING SIZE: 2
CALORIES: 336 / NET CARBS: 2G / FIBRE: 0G / FAT: 26G / PROTEIN: 23G

INGREDIENTS:

- 2 spring onions, sliced finely
- 150g //5oz chorizo, bacon, sausage or salami, chopped into cubes
- 12 eggs
- 2tbsp pesto (red or green)
- 180g // 6oz grated cheese
- Salt and pepper

METHOD:

1. First, preheat your oven to 175 degrees celsius, or 350 degrees fahrenheit.

2. Line and grease a muffin tin with greaseproof paper.

3. Mix together the chopped up meat and finely sliced spring onion, put a table spoon of the mixture in each lined muffin cup.

4. Beat together the eggs with your chosen pesto and seasoning. Add the grated cheese and mix in well.

5. Spoon the egg mixture into each muffin cup, covering the meat and onions.

6. Bake in your preheated oven for about 20 minutes, or until the muffins have risen and began to brown and bubble on the top.

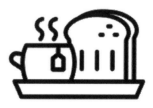

CHIA SEED PUDDING:

PREP TIME: 2 MIN / COOKING TIME: OVERNIGHT / SERVINGS: 1 / SERVING SIZE: 1
CALORIES: 568 / NET CARBS: 8G / FIBRE: 8G / FAT: 56G / PROTEIN: 9G

INGREDIENTS:

- 225ml // 1 cup of your favorite unsweetened plant milk - we recommend coconut or almond
- 25g // 2tbsp chia seeds
- ½ tsp vanilla extract
- ½ tsp cinnamon (optional)
- Fresh berries, almond butter or our keto-friendly raspberry jam to serve

METHOD:

1. Mix everything together in a glass bowl or cup. It'll seem watery but that's just because the chia seeds haven't had time to absorb the moisture and gel together!

2. Cover with a little cling-film or a saucer and place in the fridge to set.

3. Serve the next morning with fresh fruit, almond butter or our keto-friendly raspberry jam.

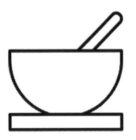

NUTTY GRANOLA:

*PREP TIME: 10 MIN / COOKING TIME: 60 MIN / SERVINGS: 10 / SERVING SIZE: ▢ CUP
CALORIES: 358 / NET CARBS: 7G / FIBRE: 5G / FAT: 29G / PROTEIN:16G*

INGREDIENTS:

- 110g // 4oz pecan nuts, hazelnuts or almonds (or a mixture of all three)
- 35g // 1 ¼ oz shredded coconut
- 75g // ½ cup sunflower seeds
- 15g // 2tbsp pumpkin seeds
- 20g // 2tbsp sesame seeds
- 75g // ⅖ cup flax seeds
- ½ turmeric
- ½ cinnamon powder
- 1tsp vanilla essence
- 30g // ¼ cup almond flour
- 125ml // ½ cup water
- 2 tbsp coconut oil
- Full-fat greek yoghurt or coconut milk to serve

METHOD:

1. First, preheat the oven to 150 degrees celsius, or 300 degrees fahrenheit.

2. Crush and chop the nuts coarsely with a sharp knife. You can choose how chunky they want them to be!

3. Mix all of the ingredients together in a large bowl. You may need to melt the coconut oil slightly if it has solidified. Simply put it in the microwave for 30 seconds to melt!

4. Spoon mixture out onto a greaseproof paper lined baking tray and spread out evenly. Bake in the oven for about 30 minutes, or until the nutty mixture is golden and crunchy. You may need to stir the mixture around every 5 minutes to help it cook evenly!

5. Once nicely browned and crunchy, turn off the oven and let the granola cool down slowly still on the oven shelf. When it's' fully cooled down you can break it apart and store in a glass or airtight container.

6. You can serve your granola with full fat coconut cream, almond milk or greek yoghurt! It's also delicious with fresh berries!

NO-NUTS KETO BREAD:

PREP TIME: 15 MIN / COOKING TIME: 35 MIN / SERVINGS: 10 / SERVING SIZE: 2 SLICES
CALORIES: 105 / NET CARBS: 1G / FIBRE: 3G / FAT: 8G / PROTEIN: 6G

INGREDIENTS:

- 3 eggs
- 175g // 6oz grated cheese
- 15g // ½ oz cream cheese
- 10g // 1tbsp ground psyllium husk powder
- 7g // 1 ½ tsp baking powder
- 25g // ¼ cup oat fiber
- ¼ tsp salt
- ½ tbsp salted butter
- 13g // 1 ½ tbsp sesame seeds
- 10g // 1tbsp poppy seeds

METHOD:

1. Preheat your oven to 180 degrees celsius, 360 degrees fahrenheit.

2. In a large bowl, beat the eggs together and add all of the ingredients apart from the butter. Mix well till everything forms a loose sticky dough.

3. Use the butter to grease and line a small bread pan, or alternatively use a muffin tray if you want little bread rolls.

4. Using a big spoon or spatula, scrape out the dough mixture into your prepared bread tin or tray. Sprinkle the seeds on top, and an additional sprinkle of sea salt and pepper.

5. Bake in the preheated oven for 35 minutes, or a little less if using a muffin tin.

6. Once risen slightly and nicely browned on the top remove from the oven and let cool! You can use this bread for almost everything! It's delicious toasted with butter, or made into a bacon sandwich for breakfast!

KETO FRENCH TOAST

MUG BREAD:

PREP TIME: 3 MIN / COOKING TIME: 3 MIN / SERVINGS: 2 / SERVING SIZE: 1
CALORIES:294 / NET CARBS: 3G / FIBRE: 4G / FAT: 27G / PROTEIN:9G

INGREDIENTS:

- 1tsp butter
- 15g // 2tbsp almond flour
- 15g // 2tbsp coconut flour
- 7g // 1 ½ tsp baking powder
- 1 pinch of salt
- 2 eggs
- 2tbsp double cream

METHOD:

1. For the mug bread, use an appropriate microwave safe mug or bowl! Grease your dish with the butter.

2. Mix all of the ingredients together in the mug with a fork, whisking until all the lumps are gone.

3. Microwave the mug bread on a high setting for around two minutes. You can insert a knife into the middle to check it's cooked all the way through. If it isn't, put it back in the microwave for another 30 seconds.

4. Let your mug bread cool for a few minutes and then carefully go round the edges with a knife. If you used enough butter it should turn out easily! You can slice your bread in half, or in quarters depending on how thin you like your slices.

FRENCH TOAST BATTER:

PREP TIME: 5 MIN / COOKING TIME: 5 MIN / SERVINGS: 2 / SERVING SIZE: 1
CALORIES:416 / NET CARBS: 4G / FIBRE: 4G / FAT: 37G / PROTEIN:15G

INGREDIENTS:

- ◆ 2 eggs
- ◆ 2 tbsp double cream
- ◆ 1 pinch salt
- ◆ 2 tbsp butter

METHOD:

1. For the french toast, whisk together the eggs, double cream and pinch of salt. At this stage you can add a little cinnamon for sweet, or grated cheese and herbs for savory.

2. Soak the slices of mug bread in the egg mixture until fully saturated, the bread will become very soggy, so take care not to break it!

3. Fry the french toast in butter for 1-2 minutes each side until cooked through and golden brown. Serve immediately while it's still hot!

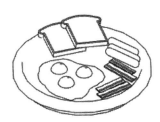

MEXICAN BREAKFAST EGGS:

PREP TIME:15 MIN / COOKING TIME: 45 MIN / SERVINGS: 4 / SERVING SIZE: 1
CALORIES: 542 / NET CARBS: 12G / FIBRE: 7G / FAT: 46G / PROTEIN: 17G

INGREDIENTS:

- 125ml // ½ cup olive oil
- 1 white onion
- 2 garlic cloves
- 2 fresh jalapenos
- 475ml // 2 cups canned diced tomatoes
- 8 eggs
- 50g // 2oz grated cheese
- 4 tbsp chopped coriander
- 1 avocado
- Pinch of salt and pepper

METHOD:

1. Finely chop the onion, garlic and jalapenos and mix together.

2. In a frying pan, add a little olive oil and sweat the onion mix to release the flavours and spices. Cook until the jalapeno becomes tender and the onions become translucent.

3. Pour over the chopped tomatoes and stir to combine. Let everything simmer for 10 minutes until the sauce becomes rich and thick. Season with a little salt and pepper, then set aside.

4. Add the remaining oil to another pan and fry each egg on a high heat so that the edges are crispy while the egg yolk is still runny.

5. Carefully place the cooked eggs on top of the tomato sauce mixture, top with cheese and place under a grill for 5 minutes, or until the cheese has melted.

6. Serve sprinkled with chopped fresh coriander and a slice or two of our keto-friendly bread.

BACON AND EGG BREAKFAST CUPS:

PREP TIME: 5 MIN / COOKING TIME: 15 MIN / SERVINGS: 3 / SERVING SIZE: 2 EGGS PER SERVE
CALORIES: 171 / NET CARBS: 1G / FIBRE: 0G / FAT: 11G / PROTEIN: 16G

INGREDIENTS:

- 75g // 3oz streaky bacon
- 75g // 3oz grated cheddar cheese
- 6 large eggs
- Pinch of salt and pepper

METHOD:

1. Preheat your oven to 200 degrees celsius, or 400 degrees fahrenheit.

2. Chop the strips of bacon in half and use them to line a 6 hole muffin pan. We use two pieces of bacon layered up and crossed over to fully line each hole.

3. Place a tablespoon of grated cheese in each hole, on top of the bacon. Then gently crack a whole egg on top of the cheese.

4. Sprinkle with a little seasoning and bake for 15 minutes, or until you can see that the egg whites have set.

BOILED EGGS WITH ASPARAGUS DIPPERS:

PREP TIME: 2 MIN / COOKING TIME: 10 MIN / SERVINGS: 2 / SERVING SIZE: 1
CALORIES: 316 / NET CARBS: 1G / FIBRE: 1G / FAT: 29G / PROTEIN:11G

INGREDIENTS:
- ♦ 4 eggs
- ♦ 4 tsp salted butter
- ♦ 10 stems of asparagus

METHOD:

1. Fill a deep cooking pot with water and bring to the boil.

2. Once at a rolling boil, turn down the temperature and carefully add your eggs with a spoon, one at a time. Be careful not to drop the eggs as you may splash yourself with boiling water.

3. Boil the eggs for 5 minutes for soft boiled (recommended) or 8 minutes for hard boiled.

4. Remove the eggs from the water with a slotted spoon and set to one side to cool slightly.

5. Using the same boiling water, place a steamer or sieve over the pan and place in your trimmed asparagus. Steam for 5-8 minutes until the asparagus is tender, but still has a slight crunch.

6. Melt the butter in the microwave and place in a small ramekin to be used as a dipping sauce.

7. Serve the eggs in egg cups with the top sliced off. You can drizzle the butter over the asparagus and dunk the stems in the runny egg yolks! Delicious!

WAYNE A. COLE

CLASSIC BACON AND EGGS:

PREP TIME: 2 MIN / COOKING TIME:10 MIN / SERVINGS: 2 / SERVING SIZE: 1
CALORIES: 272 / NET CARBS: 1G / FIBRE: 0G / FAT: 22G / PROTEIN: 15G

INGREDIENTS:

- 4 eggs
- 75g // 2 ½ oz streaky bacon
- 6 cherry tomatoes (optional)

- Bunch of fresh parsley
- Pinch of salt and pepper

METHOD:

1. Fry the bacon on a medium-high heat for 5 minutes, until it is becoming crispy.

2. Set the bacon to one side and in the same pan, add the cherry tomatoes and fry for a further 3 minutes. Set aside with the bacon.

3. Again, in the same pan, crack your eggs and fry for a further 2-3 minutes until you have the perfect runny eggs.

4. Serve together, sprinkled with fresh chopped parsley and season to taste.

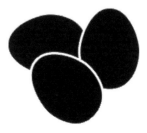

SMOOTHIES AND BREAKFAST DRINKS

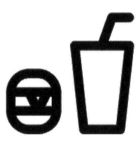

SPICED PUMPKIN LATTE:

PREP TIME: 1 MIN / COOKING TIME: 5 MIN / SERVINGS: 1 / SERVING SIZE: 1
CALORIES: 216 / NET CARBS: 1G / FIBRE: 1G / FAT: 23G / PROTEIN: 0.5G

INGREDIENTS:
- 30g // 1oz unsalted butter
- 1tsp ground pumpkin pie spice
- 2tsp unsweetened instant coffee powder
- 225ml // 1 cup hot water
- 1tbsp whipped double cream

METHOD:
1. In a blender or smoothie maker, add the instant coffee, spices and butter.

2. Pour over the hot (but not boiling) water and blend for 30-60 seconds until the latte is frothy and the instant coffee powder is fully dissolved.

3. Serve your warm latte with a generous dollop of whipped double cream and a dusting of pumpkin spice.

HOMEMADE ELECTROLYTE LEMONADE:

PREP TIME: 5 MIN / COOKING TIME: 0 MIN / SERVINGS: 2 / SERVING SIZE: 1
CALORIES: 7 / NET CARBS: 3G / FIBRE: 0G / FAT: 0G / PROTEIN: 0G

INGREDIENTS:
- 2l // 8 cups water
- 1tsp sea salt
- ½ tsp magnesium powder
- 125ml // ½ cup lemon juice
- 3 lemons, sliced
- ice

METHOD:
1. Dissolve sea salt and magnesium in a jug of water. Pour in the lemon juice.

2. Slice the 3 lemons thinly and place in the jug to infuse. Top up with ice and enjoy!

SUPER-GREENS BREAKFAST SMOOTHIE:

PREP TIME: 5 MIN / COOKING TIME: 0 MIN / SERVINGS: 2 / SERVING SIZE: 1
CALORIES: 82 / NET CARBS: 3G / FIBRE: 1G / FAT: 8G / PROTEIN: 1G

INGREDIENTS:

- 75ml // ⅓ cup coconut milk
- 150ml // ⅔ cup water
- 2tbsp lime juice
- 30g // 1oz frozen spinach
- 2tsp grated ginger

METHOD:

1. Place all ingredients into a smoothie maker or blender with ice. Blend on the high setting until smooth and frothy.

2. Sprinkle with lime zest and a little grated ginger.

FLAVOURED WATER:

PREP TIME: 2 MIN / COOKING TIME: 0 MIN / SERVINGS: 2 / SERVING SIZE: 1
CALORIES: 0 / NET CARBS: 0G / FIBRE: 0G / FAT: 0G / PROTEIN:0G

INGREDIENTS:

- 1l // 4 cups fresh, cold water
- Your desired flavoring - mint, cucumber, lemon, or summer berries work really well
- 475ml // 2 cups ice cubes

METHOD:

1. Fill a large jug with water, place your desired flavorings inside and top up with ice. Let infuse for 10 minutes in the fridge and enjoy! This flavoured water stores well for up to 2 days, and will deepen in flavour the longer you leave it.

THIRST QUENCHING ICE TEA:

PREP TIME: 5 MIN / COOKING TIME: 0 MIN / SERVINGS: 2 / SERVING SIZE: 1
CALORIES: 0G / NET CARBS: 0G / FIBRE: 0G / FAT: 0G / PROTEIN: 0G

INGREDIENTS:
- 475ml // 2 cups water
- 1 green tea bag or loose tea
- 225ml // 1 cup ice cubes
- 2 tsp sliced root ginger
- 1 lime, sliced
- 1 bunch of fresh mint leaves

METHOD:

1. Using ½ cup of hot water, brew the tea or tea bag in a heat proof mug or teapot.

2. Slice the root ginger, lime and place in a large glass jug with the stems of fresh mint.

3. Pour over the hot infused green tea. Top up with the remaining cold water.

4. Add the ice cubes and stir. This ice tea keeps really well in the fridge for up to 2 days, and will increase in flavour the longer you leave it.

CLASSIC COFFEE WITH CREAM:

PREP TIME: 5 MIN / COOKING TIME: 0 MIN / SERVINGS: 2 / SERVING SIZE: 1
CALORIES: 203G / NET CARBS: 2G / FIBRE: 0G / FAT: 21G / PROTEIN: 2G

INGREDIENTS:
- 175ml // ¾ cup black coffee, brewed to your preferred method.
- 60ml // ¼ cup double cream

METHOD:

1. Brew your coffee as you like it and serve with double cream - Either poured in and stirred, or whipped and dolloped on top!

KETO FRIENDLY HOT CHOCOLATE:

PREP TIME: 1 MIN / COOKING TIME: 3 MIN / SERVINGS: 1 / SERVING SIZE: 1
CALORIES: 300 / NET CARBS: 12G / FIBRE: 2G / FAT: 23G / PROTEIN: 5G

INGREDIENTS:

- 30g salted butter
- 5g // 1tbsp cocoa powder
- 10g // 2 ½ tsp powdered erythritol
- ¼ tsp vanilla extract
- 225ml full cream milk.

METHOD:

1. Combine all ingredients in a large heavy base saucepan.

2. Gently bring to the boil, whisking all the time until all ingredients are combined.

3. Serve in mugs. Tastes delicious with a dollop of whipped cream and a dusting of cocoa.

BLUEBERRY BREAKFAST SMOOTHIE:

PREP TIME: 5 MIN / COOKING TIME: 0 MIN / SERVINGS: 2 / SERVING SIZE: 1
CALORIES: 417 / NET CARBS: 10G / FIBRE: 1G / FAT: 43G / PROTEIN: 4G

INGREDIENTS:

- 400g // 14oz coconut milk
- 75g // 3oz frozen blueberries
- 1tbsp lemon juice
- ½ tsp vanilla essence

METHOD:

1. Combine all ingredients in a smoothie maker and blend for 30-60 seconds until smooth and frothy.

WAYNE A. COLE

VANILLA ICE LATTE

PREP TIME: 5 MIN / COOKING TIME: 0 MIN / SERVINGS: 2 / SERVING SIZE: 1
CALORIES: 203G / NET CARBS: 2G / FIBRE: 0G / FAT: 21G / PROTEIN: 2G

INGREDIENTS:
- 175ml // ¾ cup black coffee, brewed to your preferred method.
- 60ml // ¼ cup double cream
- ½ tsp vanilla extract
- Ice cubes

METHOD:
1. Brew your coffee as you like it and pour over ice. Stir in the vanilla extract.
2. Serve with whipped double cream dolloped on top!

STRAWBERRY MILKSHAKE:

PREP TIME: 5 MIN / COOKING TIME: 0 MIN / SERVINGS: 2 / SERVING SIZE: 1
CALORIES: 210G / NET CARBS: 1G / FIBRE: 0G / FAT: 25G / PROTEIN: 2G

INGREDIENTS:
- 400g // 14oz coconut milk
- 150g // 5oz fresh strawberries
- ½ tsp vanilla essence
- 100ml // ½ cup ice cubes
- Dollop of whipped cream on top

METHOD:
1. Put all ingredients in a smoothie maker and blend on high power for five minutes.
2. Serve with whipped cream on top.

LUNCH

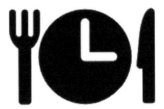

CHEESY CROQUE MADAME:

PREP TIME: 10 MIN / COOKING TIME: 15 MIN / SERVINGS: 2 / SERVING SIZE: 1
CALORIES: 1247 / NET CARBS: 10G / FIBRE: 5G / FAT: 107G / PROTEIN: 60G

Recipe Note: *You can make this croque madame even cheesier with the addition of a healthy dollop of our creamy keto-friendly bechamel sauce! Delicious!*

INGREDIENTS:

- 225g // 8oz cottage cheese
- 4 eggs
- 10g // 1tbsp psyllium husk powder (to thicken)
- 4tbsp salted butter
- 150g // 5oz smoked ham
- 150g // 5oz grated cheddar cheese
- ½ red onion, finely sliced
- Serving:
- 2 eggs
- 2 tbsp salted butter
- 40g // 1 ½ oz spinach
- Salt and pepper

METHOD:

1. Whisk the eggs and cottage cheese together until fully combined. Stir in the ground psyllium powder until combined smoothly with no lumps. Leave the batter for five minutes to thicken up.

2. Using a liberal amount of butter, fly the eggy batter into little pancakes over a medium heat, until golden on both sides. We will use these as a substitute for bread so allow two pancakes for each serving!

3. Create your sandwich with slices of ham and grated cheese between the warm pancakes. Thinly slice your red onion and sprinkle this on top.

4. Fry your eggs sunny-side up, and place on top of the sandwich.

5. Dress the spinach with salt, pepper and your favorite infused olive oil and serve!

MUSHROOM AND BACON SLICE:

PREP TIME: 10 MIN / COOKING TIME: 45 MIN / SERVINGS: 4 / SERVING SIZE: ¼ SLICE
CALORIES: 876 / NET CARBS: 6 / FIBRE: 1G / FAT: 81G / PROTEIN: 31G

INGREDIENTS:

- 175g // 6oz mushrooms
- 275g // 10oz streaky bacon
- 50g // 2oz butter
- 8 eggs
- 225ml // 1 cup double cream
- 150g // 5oz grated cheddar cheese
- 1tsp onion powder
- A pinch of salt and pepper

METHOD:

1. Preheat your oven to 200 degrees celsius or 400 degrees fahrenheit.

2. Slice up the mushrooms and bacon into chunky strips and fry with the butter until cooked and golden brown. Season with the salt and pepper.

3. Whisk together the eggs, double cream, cheese and onion powder.

4. Grease a casserole tray with a little butter. Sprinkle in the cooked mushrooms and bacon and arrange evenly in the tray.

5. Pour over your egg mixture, cover with tin foil and bake in the preheated oven for 30-40 minutes until cooked all the way through and golden brown!

6. This breakfast slice can be served hot or cold!

CRISPY KALE AND BACON BOWL WITH A FRIED EGG:

PREP TIME: 5 MIN / COOKING TIME: 20 MIN / SERVINGS: 2 / SERVING SIZE: 1
CALORIES: 384 / NET CARBS: 10G / FIBRE:6G / FAT: 28G / PROTEIN: 20G

INGREDIENTS:
- 110g // 4oz streaky bacon
- 325g // 3/4lb kale
- 2 eggs
- Pinch of salt and pepper

METHOD:
1. Slice up the bacon into small chunks and pan-fry for a few minutes, until crispy and the fat has become golden. Set the bacon pieces aside.

2. Wash, dry and shred the kale leaves with a sharp knife and add to the same pan as the bacon. Fly in the bacon fat until the leaves are wilted, then season with a little salt and pepper.

3. Fry the eggs sunny-side up in the same hot frying pan.

4. Serve the eggs on a bed of kale and crispy bacon! Add some cracked black pepper on top!

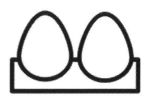

SPINACH FRITTATA:

PREP TIME: 10 MIN / COOKING TIME: 35 MIN / SERVINGS: 4 / SERVING SIZE: 1 SLICE
CALORIES: 661 / NET CARBS: 4G / FIBRE: 1G / FAT: 59G / PROTEIN: 27G

INGREDIENTS:
- ◆ 150g // 5oz chorizo sausage
- ◆ 2tbsp butter
- ◆ 225g // 8oz spinach
- ◆ 8 eggs
- ◆ 225ml // 1 cup double cream
- ◆ 150g // 5oz grated cheddar cheese
- ◆ Pinch of salt and pepper

METHOD:
1. Preheat your oven to 175 degrees celsius, or 350 degrees fahrenheit.
2. Fry the chopped chorizo sausage with the butter to let release the oils. When crispy, add the spinach and fry together until wilted. Season with salt and pepper and set aside.
3. Beat together the eggs and double cream.
4. Grease a shallow baking dish and pour in the egg mixture. Arrange the crispy chorizo sausage, wilted spinach and grated cheese on the top.
5. Bake in the pre heated oven for 30 minutes until the frittata is fully set in the middle, and the cheese on the top is golden brown.

CLOUD BREAD:

PREP TIME: 25 MIN / COOKING TIME: 20 MIN / SERVINGS: 2 / SERVING SIZE: 1
CALORIES: 162 / NET CARBS: 2GG / FIBRE: 1G / FAT: 14G / PROTEIN: 6G

INGREDIENTS:

- 3 eggs
- 110g // 4oz cream cheese
- 5g // ½ tbsp ground psyllium husk powder
- 2.5g // ½ tsp baking powder

METHOD:

1. Preheat your oven to 150 degrees celsius, or 300 degrees fahrenheit.

2. Carefully separate the eggs. The whites in a big mixing bowl, and the yolks set aside in a cup to be used later.

3. Whisk the egg whites thoroughly for 5-10 minutes, ideally with an electric mixer if you have ones. The whites need to be standing up in stiff peaks when you are finished.

4. Beat together the cream cheese, psyllium husk powder, egg yolks and baking powder.

5. Using a spatula, gently fold the egg yolk mixture into the stiff egg whites, do this gently to keep as much air in the egg whites as possible.

6. Grease and line a baking tray with greaseproof paper. Dollop big spoonfuls of the egg mixture onto the tray and use the back of the spoon to flatten them to about 1cm thick.

7. Bake in the preheated oven for 30 minutes, until the cloud bread is turning a golden colour. Set aside to cool while you make your sandwich filling.

BACON, LETTUCE AND TOMATO SANDWICHES (WITH CLOUD BREAD):

PREP TIME: 10 MIN / COOKING TIME: 5 MIN / SERVINGS: 2 / SERVING SIZE: 1
CALORIES: 800 / NET CARBS: 7G / FIBRE: 3G / FAT: 75G / PROTEIN: 22G

INGREDIENTS:

- 4tbsp mayonnaise
- 150g // 5oz bacon
- 50g // 2oz lettuce
- 1 tomato, thinly sliced
- Cloud bread

METHOD:

1. Fry the bacon until it's crispy and golden and then set aside.

2. Spread mayonnaise on each piece of cloud bread, and then assemble your sandwich with layers of crispy bacon, crunchy fresh lettuce and thinly sliced tomato. Enjoy!

CHEESE AND RED ONION SANDWICH WITH CLOUD BREAD:

PREP TIME: 5 MIN / COOKING TIME: 0 MIN / SERVINGS: 2 / SERVING SIZE: 1
CALORIES: 800 / NET CARBS: 7G / FIBRE: 3G / FAT: 75G / PROTEIN: 22G

INGREDIENTS:

- 150g // 5oz cheddar cheese
- ¼ red onion
- 1tbsp mayonnaise
- Cloud bread

METHOD:

1. Grate the cheese and thinly slice the red onion.

2. Spread mayonnaise on each side of the cloud bread and assemble your sandwich.

NO BAKE SALMON AND AVOCADO BOATS:

PREP TIME: 5 MIN / COOKING TIME: 0 MIN / SERVINGS: 2 / SERVING SIZE: 1
CALORIES:717 / NET CARBS: 6G / FIBRE:13G / FAT: 65G / PROTEIN: 22G

INGREDIENTS:

- 2 ripe avocados
- 175g // 6oz smoked salmon
- 175g // ¾ cup creme fraiche or sour cream
- ½ a lemon
- Pinch of salt and pepper
- Chopped parsley

METHOD:

1. Cut the avocados in half and carefully remove the pit, you can leave the skin on, this creates our little boats.

2. Spoon a generous dollop of creme fraiche or sour cream into the hollow, left by the avocado pit.

3. Place strips of salmon decretavly on top, then garnish with chopped parsley and a wedge of fresh lemon. Season to taste with the salt and pepper.

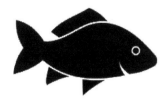

TUNA PLATE:

PREP TIME: 5 MIN / COOKING TIME: 10 MIN / SERVINGS: 2 / SERVING SIZE: 1
CALORIES: 931 / NET CARBS: 3G / FIBRE: 7G / FAT: 76G / PROTEIN: 52G

INGREDIENTS:

- 4 eggs
- 50g // 2oz baby spinach
- 257g // 10oz canned tuna, in oil
- 1 avocado

- 125ml // ½ cup mayonnaise
- ¼ lemon
- Pinch of salt and pepper

METHOD:

1. First, boil the eggs in a large saucepan for between 4-8 minutes depending on how you like them, soft or hard. Once cooked, remove from the boiling water and submerge in a bowl of ice water. This will help the eggs stop cooking, and make it easier to remove the shell.

2. Slice the avocado in half and remove the pit and the skin. Slice into neat strips.

3. Arrange the baby spinach and avocado on a plate.

4. Remove shells from the eggs and cut each into quarters.

5. Arrange eggs and tuna on the bed of spinach and avocado. Place a large dollop of mayonnaise on the side and garnish with a few wedges of lemon. Season with salt and pepper according to your tastes.

BAKED GOATS CHEESE SALAD:

PREP TIME: 5 MIN / COOKING TIME: 10 MIN / SERVINGS: 2 / SERVING SIZE: 1
CALORIES: 824 / NET CARBS: 3G / FIBRE: 2G / FAT: 73G / PROTEIN: 37G

INGREDIENTS:
- 275g // 10oz goats cheese
- 35g // ¼ cups pumpkin seeds
- 50g // 2oz butter
- 1tbsp balsamic vinegar
- 75g // 3oz baby spinach

METHOD:
1. Preheat your oven to 200 degrees celsius, or 400 degrees fahrenheit.

2. Slice the goats cheese and lay out on a greased baking tray. Bake in the oven for 10 minutes.

3. While the goat's cheese is baking, toast the pumpkin seeds in a dry frying pan. They should begin to pop and change colour.

4. Lower the heat and add butter to the pumpkin seeds, the butter will begin to brown and take on a lovely rich nutty flavour.

5. Add the balsamic vinegar to the pumpkin seeds and butter and simmer for a few minutes to reduce.

6. Wash and dry the baby spinach, then lay out on a plate. Using a spatula remove the warm goats cheese from the baking tray and lay on top of the spinach.

7. Dress the salad with the warm pumpkin and balsamic dressing and serve.

PRAWN DEVILED EGGS:

PREP TIME: 5 MIN / COOKING TIME: 10 MIN / SERVINGS: 4 / SERVING SIZE: 1
CALORIES: 163 / NET CARBS: 0.5G / FIBRE: 0G / FAT: 15G / PROTEIN: 7G

INGREDIENTS:

- 4eggs
- 1tsp tabasco
- 60ml // ¼ cup mayonnaise
- 8 cooked and peeled king prawns
- Bunch of fresh dill
- Pinch of salt and pepper
- ¼ lemon

METHOD:

1. Begin by boiling the eggs in a large saucepan of water. To ensure the eggs are hard-boiled, cook them for 8-10 minutes. Once the eggs are done, transfer to a bowl of ice water to let them cool.

2. Once the eggs have cooled, peel and half them. Using a teaspoon, gently scoop out the yolks and arrange the whites on a plate.

3. Mash the leftover egg yolks with the tabasco, salt, pepper and mayonnaise.

4. Gently spoon the yolk mixture back into the egg white sections.

5. Place the cooked and peeled king prawns on each egg half and garnish with fresh dill and a few wedges of lemon.

CAESAR SALAD:

PREP TIME: 12 MIN / COOKING TIME: 20 MIN / SERVINGS: 2 / SERVING SIZE: 1
CALORIES: 1018 / NET CARBS: 4G / FIBRE: 3G / FAT: 87G / PROTEIN: 51G

INGREDIENTS:

- ¾ lb chicken breast
- 1 tbsp olive oil
- 3oz bacon
- 7oz lettuce, such as romaine or iceberg
- 1oz parmesan cheese, thinly sliced or shaven
- 4 tbsp caesar dressing (see recipe)

METHOD:

1. Fry the chicken breast with a little olive oil over a medium heat, when the chicken is thoroughly cooked all the way through, take it off the heat and let it cool.

2. Fry the bacon in the same hot pan until it's crispy.

3. Wash and dry the lettuce leaves and arrange on a plate. Top with the sliced up chicken breast, crispy bacon pieces, and parmesan cheese.

4. Spoon the dressing over the salad and garnish with shavings of parmesan cheese.

CREAMY CAULIFLOWER SALAD:

PREP TIME: 10 MIN / COOKING TIME: 25 MIN / SERVINGS: 6 / SERVING SIZE: 1
CALORIES: 512 / NET CARBS: 5G / FIBRE: 3G / FAT: 51G / PROTEIN: 6G

INGREDIENTS:

- 700g // 25oz cauliflower head
- 125ml // ½ cup water
- 150g // 5oz streaky bacon
- 3 celery sticks
- ½ red onion
- 2tbsp chopped fresh chives
- 12 tbsp creamy mustard vinaigrette salad dressing (see recipe)
- Pinch of salt and pepper

METHOD:

1. Chop the cauliflower and bacon into bite-sized chunks. Steam the cauliflower over a pan of boiling water for 10 minutes, or until soft. Once cooked, leave to one side to cool.

2. Fry the bacon with a little oil until crispy and set aside to cool.

3. Chop the onion, celery and chives into small pieces.

4. Combine all ingredients in a bowl and season to taste with salt and pepper.

5. Pour the dressing over the salad and toss to fully combine all the pieces in dressing.

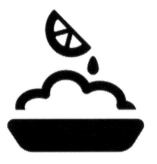

CRUNCHY WALNUT AND COURGETTE SALAD:

PREP TIME: 20 MIN / COOKING TIME: 15 MIN / SERVINGS: 4 / SERVING SIZE: 1
CALORIES: 595 / NET CARBS: 8G / FIBRE: 7G / FAT: 58G / PROTEIN: 9G

INGREDIENTS:

- 1 large head of lettuce, such as iceberg or romaine
- 6 finely chopped spring onions
- 2 medium sized courgettes (or 4 baby ones)
- 1tbsp olive oil
- 100g // 3 ½ oz walnuts, roughly chopped
- 8 tbsp very versatile creamy salad dressing (see recipe)
- Pinch of salt and pepper

METHOD:

1. Wash and dry the lettuce leaves. Roughly chop the leaves and place in a serving bowl. Scatter over the chopped spring onions.

2. Slice the courgettes long-ways, scoop out the seeds in the middle and chop roughly into bite sized pieces.

3. Heat the olive oil in a pan and add the courgette pieces. Fry on both sides until the courgette is cooked and takes on a lovely golden brown colour on the outside, but is still firm. Season with salt and pepper and put to one side to cool a little.

4. Add the warm courgette pieces to the salad and toss to incorporate.

5. Spoon on the dressing and scatter the salad with roughly chopped walnuts.

TRADITIONAL NICOISE SALAD:

PREP TIME: 15 MIN / COOKING TIME: 10 MIN / SERVINGS: 2 / SERVING SIZE: 1
CALORIES: 957 / NET CARBS: 11G / FIBRE:6G / FAT: 85G / PROTEIN: 34G

INGREDIENTS:

- 2 eggs
- 50g // 2oz turnip
- 150 // 5oz crunchy green beans
- 2tbsp olive oil
- 2 garlic cloves
- 150 // 5oz lettuce leaves
- 50g // 2oz cherry tomatoes, halved
- ½ red onion, sliced thinly
- 1 can of tuna in olive oil
- 50g // 2oz black pitted olives
- 4 tbsp nicoise dressing (see recipe)
- Pinch of salt and pepper

METHOD:

1. In a large pan of water, boil your eggs the way you like them. 5 minutes for soft boiled or 8-10 for hard boiled. Once the eggs are cooked, transfer them to a bowl of ice water to cool them down. Peel and cut the boiled eggs into quarters one cooled.

2. Top and tail the green beans, and peel the turnip. Cut everything into 1-2 inch pieces and boil (or steam) for 5 minutes until cooked, but still retaining some crunch. Set aside to cool.

3. Transfer the green beans to a frying pan. Lightly fry with olive oil and garlic and season with salt and pepper.

4. Place washed lettuce leaves on a plate and decorate with green beans and cooked turnip. Add tuna, sliced eggs, cherry tomatoes, sliced red onion and black olives. Spoon over the nicoise dressing and serve!

BAKED SALMON WITH CREAMY PESTO DRESSING:

PREP TIME: 5 MIN / COOKING TIME: 15 MIN / SERVINGS: 4 / SERVING SIZE: 1
CALORIES: 1025 / NET CARBS: 3G / FIBRE: G / FAT: 88G / PROTEIN: 52G

INGREDIENTS:
- 900g // 2lb salmon fillet
- 4tbsp green pesto
- Pinch of salt and pepper
- Sauce:
- 4tbsp green pesto
- 225ml // 1 cup mayonnaise
- 125ml // ½ cup green yoghurt
- Pinch of salt and pepper

METHOD:
1. Preheat the grill. Put the salmon skin side down on an aluminum foil lined baking tray.

2. Season the fish and spread a little green pesto on the top. Drizzle with olive oil and grill for about 20 minutes, until the pesto on the top is looking browned and a little crispy.

3. For the sauce, mix together the remaining ingredients in a bowl and whisk until blended.

4. Serve the fish flaked over a bed of crunchy salad, with courgette noodles, or accompanying steamed green veggies.

TOMATO AND PARMASAN SOUP:

PREP TIME: 5 MIN / COOKING TIME: 15 MIN / SERVINGS: 12 / SERVING SIZE: 1
CALORIES: 146 / NET CARBS: 3G / FIBRE: 1G / FAT: 12G / PROTEIN: 6G

INGREDIENTS:

- 2tbsp butter
- 110g // 4oz red onion
- 2 garlic cloves
- 1tbsp dried basil
- 1tsp dried oregano
- 225g // 8oz cream cheese or sour cream
- 1l // 4 cups chicken stock
- 2 cans of chopped tomatoes
- 150g // 5oz grated parmesan
- 1tsp salt
- 1tsp black pepper
- 4-6 fresh basil leaves as a garnish

METHOD:

1. Chop the onions and garlic and add to a large pot. Saute in butter for a few minutes until the onion becomes soft and translucent. Add the dried herbs and stir.

2. Add the cream cheese (or sour cream) to the pot and slowly stir until it softens and mixes with the onion and herbs.

3. Gradually add the chicken stock, a cup at a time, stirring as you go to incorporate the cream cheese.

4. Pour in the two tins of chopped tomatoes, grated parmesan cheese and seasoning. Let simmer for 5 minutes.

5. Once the soup is thickening up to the desired consistency, transfer into a food processor and blend for 2 minutes until creamy and smooth. If the soup is still a little thin you can put it back on the hob for a further 5 minutes to simmer and reduce.

6. Serve in bowls garnished with fresh basil leaves and an extra grating of parmesan cheese. This soup is delicious with a slice or two of our keto-friendly bread.

WINTER WARMER CHICKEN SOUP:

PREP TIME: 10 MIN / COOKING TIME: 20 MIN / SERVINGS: 8 / SERVING SIZE: 1
CALORIES: 519 / NET CARBS: 4G / FIBRE: 1G / FAT: 40G / PROTEIN: 33G

INGREDIENTS:

- 110g // 4oz butter
- 2tbsp white onion, chopped
- 2 celery sticks, chopped
- 175g // 6oz mushrooms, chopped
- 2 garlic cloves, minced
- 1 bay leaf
- 2l // 8 cups chicken stock
- 1 medium carrot, chopped
- 2tsp dried parsley
- 4 pre-cooked chicken breasts
- 150g // 5oz green cabbage, chopped

METHOD:

1. Chop and dice all of the vegetables into neat little chunks or strips. In a large pot, saute the vegetables in butter over a medium heat for 5 minutes until they begin to soften.

2. Add the dried parsley and bayleaf. Pour over the chicken stock and let simmer for 5 minutes.

3. Shred the cooked (roasted, fried or boiled) chicken breasts with two forks. Add the chicken to the pot and continue simmering for a further 10 minutes, or until the vegetables are tender.

4. Remember to remove the bay-leaf before serving.

5. Serve with a sprinkle of parsley and a few slices of our delicious keto-friendly bread.

CREAMY BROCCOLI AND LEEK SOUP:

PREP TIME: 5 MIN / COOKING TIME: 15 MIN / SERVINGS: 4 / SERVING SIZE: 1
CALORIES:545 / NET CARBS: 10G / FIBRE: 3G / FAT: 50G / PROTEIN: 15G

INGREDIENTS:

- 1 medium leek
- 300g // ⅔ lb broccoli
- 475ml // 2 cups of water
- 1 vegetable stock cube
- 200g // 7oz cream cheese
- 225ml // 1 cup double cream
- ½ tsp chopped fresh basil
- 1 garlic clove, minced
- Pinch of salt and pepper

METHOD:

1. Wash and chop the leek and broccoli into small chunks.

2. Place vegetables in a large pot, pour over the water and add the stock cube, garlic and seasoning. Bring to the boil and simmer until the broccoli stems are soft.

3. Pour in the double cream and cream cheese and then stir until fully combined.

4. Transfer soup to a food processor and blend for 60 seconds, or until the soup is creamy and smooth.

5. Serve the soup in bowls, scattered with fresh basil.

CHICKEN WINGS WITH CHIPOTLE AIOLI:

PREP TIME: 10 MIN / COOKING TIME: 40 MIN / SERVINGS: 4 / SERVING SIZE: 1
CALORIES: 569 / NET CARBS: 2G / FIBRE: 1G / FAT: 42G / PROTEIN: 42G

INGREDIENTS:
- 900g // 2lb chicken wings (or thighs/ drumsticks)
- 2tbsp olive oil
- 2tbsp tomato paste
- 1tsp salt
- 1tsp paprika powder
- 1tbsp chipotle tabasco (or other spicy sauce)
- Chipotle Aioli dip (see recipe)

METHOD:

1. Mix together the olive oil, tomato paste, salt, paprika powder and tabasco to make a marinade. Coat the chicken wings liberally in marinade and set to one side to infuse for 10-20 minutes.

2. While the chicken is marinating, preheat the oven to 220 degrees celsius, or 450 degrees fahrenheit.

3. Bake the chicken wings on a baking tray in the middle of the oven for 30 minutes, until they're thoroughly cooked.

4. Serve the wings with Chipotle Aioli dip.

DINNER

WAYNE A. COLE

PAN FRIED CHICKEN BREAST WITH HERB BUTTER:

PREP TIME: 10 MIN / COOKING TIME: 10 MIN / SERVINGS: 4 / SERVING SIZE: 1
CALORIES: 898 / NET CARBS: 2G / FIBRE: 2G / FAT: 70G / PROTEIN: 63G

INGREDIENTS:

- 3tbsp butter
- 4 chicken breasts
- Pinch of salt and pepper
- 225g // 8oz green vegetables, such as broccoli or kale
- Herb Butter (see recipes)

METHOD:

1. Start by melting the butter in a large frying pan over a medium heat. Sprinkle salt and pepper seasoning over the chicken breast and place in the frying pan.

2. Cook the chicken till it's thoroughly cooked through and registers at 75 degrees celsius in the middle with a meat thermometer.

3. Using the same pan, sautee the green veggies until cooked through.

4. Serve the chicken on a bed of green vegetables with a generous dollop of herb butter.

PORK, ONION AND GREEN PEPPER STIR FRY:

PREP TIME: 5 MIN / COOKING TIME: 15 MIN / SERVINGS: 2 / SERVING SIZE: 1
CALORIES: 872 / NET CARBS: 5G / FIBRE: 4G / FAT: 81G / PROTEIN: 31G

INGREDIENTS:

- 110g // 4oz butter
- 300g // ⅓ lb pork, cut into strips
- 2 large green peppers, cut into strips
- 5 spring onions, cut into 1 inch pieces
- 1tsp chilli paste
- 30g // 1oz cashew nuts
- Pinch of salt and pepper

METHOD:

1. Fry the pork strips in butter over a high heat until browning nicely.

2. Add the strips of green pepper and spring onion pieces and continue to fry.

3. Throw in the cashew nuts, chilli paste and salt and pepper.

4. Once everythings nicely browned, remove from the heat and serve in a bowl with additional melted butter drizzled on top.

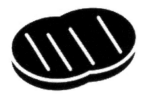

INDIAN CHICKEN KORMA CURRY:

PREP TIME: 15 MIN / COOKING TIME: 30 MIN / SERVINGS: 4 / SERVING SIZE: 1
CALORIES: 446 / NET CARBS: 4G / FIBRE: 1G / FAT: 31G / PROTEIN: 34G

INGREDIENTS:

- 4tbsp butter
- 1 red onion
- 110g // 4oz green yoghurt
- 3 whole cloves
- 1 bay leaf
- 1 cinnamon stick
- 1 star anise
- 3 green cardamom pods
- 8 whole black peppercorns

- 650g // 1 ½ lb chicken breast, thighs or drumsticks
- 1tsp ginger, minced
- 3 garlic cloves, minced
- 1tsp chilli powder
- 1tsp coriander powder
- ½ tsp turmeric
- 1tsp garam masala
- Pinch of salt and pepper
- Fresh coriander to garnish

METHOD:

1. Fry the sliced onions with butter in a frying pan until golden and crispy. Remove the onions from the pan and mix with the greek yoghurt. Blend together in a food processor to create a creamy paste.

2. In the same hot pan, add the cinnamon stick, bay leaf, star anise, cardamom pods and pepper corns. Fry for 1 minute to release the oils.

3. Add the chicken to the hot pan and season well. Add the minced garlic and ginger and stir to coat the chicken as it fries. Add all other herbs and spices at this stage.

4. Pour in the onion and yoghurt paste, and a little water. Stir well, simmer and cover for 20 minutes, or until the chicken is cooked through and the sauce has thickened.

5. Serve on a bed of cauliflower rice, sprinkled with fresh coriander leaves.

PORK SAUSAGES WITH CREAMY CABBAGE MASH:

PREP TIME: 5 MIN / COOKING TIME: 20 MIN / SERVINGS: 4 / SERVING SIZE: 1
CALORIES: 1276 / NET CARBS: 12G / FIBRE: 5G / FAT: 115G / PROTEIN: 46G

INGREDIENTS:

- 650g // 1 ½ lb green cabbage
- 50g // 2oz salted butter
- 350ml // 1 ½ cups double cream
- 650g good quality, gluten-free pork sausages
- Bunch of fresh parsley
- Pinch of salt and pepper

METHOD:

1. Fry the sausages in a little oil till browned on the outside and cooked all the way through.

2. Slice the cabbage thinly and saute in butter until beginning to turn golden brown.

3. Pour in the cream and add seasoning to taste. Let simmer until the cream has reduced and the cabbage is tender.

4. Serve together on a plate with a scattering of fresh parsley.

BROCCOLI AND CAULIFLOWER CHEESE WITH SAUSAGE:

PREP TIME: 15 MIN / COOKING TIME: 30 MIN / SERVINGS: 4 / SERVING SIZE: 1
CALORIES: 496 / NET CARBS: 12G / FIBRE: 4G / FAT: 42G / PROTEIN: 18G

INGREDIENTS:

- ◆ 450g // 1lb broccoli
- ◆ 450 // 1lb cauliflower
- ◆ 450g // 1lb pork sausages
- ◆ 450g // 2 cups homemade bechamel sauce (see recipe)
- ◆ 150g // 5oz grated cheese

METHOD:

1. Steam broccoli and cauliflower until tender. Mix with bechamel sauce and place in a baking dish.

2. Fry the sausages and arrange on top of the broccoli and cauliflower cheese. Spread the cheese on top and grill until the cheese melts.

KETO LASAGNA:

PREP TIME: 60 MIN / COOKING TIME: 30 MIN / SERVINGS: 6 / SERVING SIZE: 1
CALORIES: 875 / NET CARBS: 9G / FIBRE: 8G / FAT: 74G / PROTEIN: 40G

INGREDIENTS:

- 3 large courgettes
- 1 yellow onion
- 2 garlic cloves
- 650g // 1 ½ lb minced beef
- 2 tbsp olive oil
- 1tbsp dried basil
- 1tbsp dried oregano

- 4tbsp tomato paste
- 3tbsp water
- 200g // 7oz grated cheese
- 800g // 4 cups homemade bechamel sauce (see recipe)
- Pinch of salt and pepper

METHOD:

1. Preheat the oven to 200c, or 400f.

2. For the meat sauce, finely chop the onion and garlic and fry with the herbs, olive oil and minced beef until browned. Add the tomato paste and water and simmer.

3. Thinly slice the courgette longways, these will be used as your keto-friendly lasagne sheets.

4. Layer the lasagne with the meat sauce, courgette slices and homemade bechamel sauce. Top with grated cheese and bake for 20 minutes.

SCALLOPS WITH HERB BUTTER:

PREP TIME: 5 MIN / COOKING TIME: 10 MIN / SERVINGS: 4 / SERVING SIZE: 1
CALORIES: 260 / NET CARBS: 3G / FIBRE: 0G / FAT: 25G / PROTEIN: 8G

INGREDIENTS:
- ♦ 8 scallops
- ♦ 8tsp homemade herb butter (see recipe)

METHOD:

1. Fry the scallops in a skillet for 30 seconds, until nicely brown and seared.

2. Place back in the shells, add a tsp of herb butter on each scallop and bake in a hot oven for 5 minutes, until the butter begins to sizzle.

3. Serve with a side salad and keto bread, or as a starter if you plan on having more than one course.

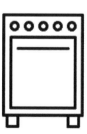

SPICY PRAWN SALAD:

PREP TIME: 5 MIN / COOKING TIME: 5 MIN / SERVINGS: 2 / SERVING SIZE: 1
CALORIES: 871 / NET CARBS: 9G / FIBRE: 16G / FAT: 79G / PROTEIN: 26G

INGREDIENTS:

- 2 avocados
- ½ lime, juiced
- 150g // 5oz cucumber
- 50g // 2oz baby spinach
- 3tbsp chilli infused olive oil
- 1 garlic clove
- 2tsp chilli powder
- 275g // 10oz peeled prawns
- Small bunch of fresh coriander to garnish

METHOD:

1. Fry the peeled prawns with a little chilli oil, chilli powder and the minced garlic till pink and begin to brown. Set aside and cool.

2. Chop the cucumber into 1cm pieces, and mix with the baby spinach in a bowl.

3. Scatter the spicy prawns over the top, drizzle with a little more chill oil and garnish with coriander.

BRUSSEL SPROUTS WITH BACON AND RED ONION:

PREP TIME: 10 MIN / COOKING TIME: 20 MIN / SERVINGS: 4 / SERVING SIZE: 1
CALORIES: 261 / NET CARBS: 8G / FIBRE: 5G / FAT: 23G / PROTEIN: 4G

INGREDIENTS:

- 1 red onion
- 110g // 4oz butter
- 1tbsp red wine vinegar
- 450g // 1lb brussel sprouts
- 150g // 5oz bacon

METHOD:

1. Fry the bacon until crispy and set to one side. Let cool and chop up into small pieces.

2. Slice the onion into small wedges and fry with butter in the same hot pan as the bacon for 5-10 minutes till soft. Add the vinegar and seasoning. Simmer for another 5 minutes.

3. Cut each brussel sprout in half and add to the pan, add the rest of the butter and fry until soft.

4. Mix in the bacon pieces and stir to incorporate.

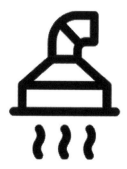

BAKED BRIE WITH WALNUTS AND ROSEMARY:

PREP TIME: 5 MIN / COOKING TIME: 10 MIN / SERVINGS: 4 / SERVING SIZE: 1
CALORIES: 342 / NET CARBS: 1G / FIBRE: 1G / FAT: 31G / PROTEIN: 15G

INGREDIENTS:

- 250g // 9oz wheel of brie
- 1 garlic clove, sliced thinly
- 1 sprig fresh rosemary
- 50g // 2oz walnuts
- 1tsp olive oil
- Pinch of salt and pepper

METHOD:

1. Preheat the oven to 200c or 400f.

2. Place the round of cheese on a baking tray lined with greaseproof paper. Using a knife score the top of the cheese in a criss cross pattern.

3. Stuff the slices of garlic and pieces of rosemary into the incisions in the cheese. Season well with salt and pepper and drizzle with olive oil.

4. Bake in the oven for 10 minutes. Remove from the oven and serve hot with chopped walnuts on top.

5. You could serve this with a selection of your favourite raw keto-friendly veggies to dip!

TURNIP GRATIN:

INGREDIENTS:

- ½ yellow onion
- 650g // 1 ½ lb turnips
- 1 garlic clove
- 125ml // ½ cup chives, chopped
- 400g // 2 cups homemade bechamel sauce (see recipe)
- 200g // 7oz grated cheese

METHOD:

1. Wash and peel the turnips then slice very finely with a sharp knife or mandolin.

2. Slice the onion very finely and fry with the garlic for a few minutes until soft.

3. Layer the turnip slices between spoonfuls of bechamel sauce. On the top layer spread out the onion and garlic mixture and grated cheese.

4. Bake in the oven at 200c or 400f for 30 minutes, or until the top is bubbling and the turnip is soft. Sprinkle with chopped chives and serve.

PORK CHOPS WITH BUTTERY GREEN BEANS:

PREP TIME: 15 MIN / COOKING TIME: 40 MIN / SERVINGS: 4 / SERVING SIZE: 1
CALORIES: 833 / NET CARBS: 6G / FIBRE: 9G / FAT: 76G / PROTEIN: 38G

INGREDIENTS:
- 800g // 1 ¾ lb pork chops
- 2tbsp olive oil
- 4tbsp homemade garlic and herb butter (see recipe)
- 300g // ⅔ lb green beans
- Pinch of salt and pepper

METHOD:
1. Place the pork chops on a baking tray, season well and brush with half of the garlic and herb butter. Bake in the oven for 20-30 minutes at 200c or 400f.

2. While the chops are in the oven, wash and trim the green beans. Place in a steamer for 15 minutes until the beans are tender.

3. Remove the pork chops from the oven and serve with the green beans. Drizzle the remaining garlic and herb butter on top.

CHICKEN AND BROCCOLI STIR FRY:

PREP TIME: 5 MIN / COOKING TIME: 10 MIN / SERVINGS: 4 / SERVING SIZE: 1
CALORIES: 753 / NET CARBS: 5G / FIBRE: 2G / FAT: 66G / PROTEIN: 32G

INGREDIENTS:
- 680g // 1.5lb chicken breast
- 2tbsp olive oil
- 1tsp garlic, minced
- 284g // 10oz broccoli
- 2tbsp soy sauce

METHOD:
1. Chop the chicken breast and broccoli into small chunks.

2. Stir fry everything in a large wok or frying pan. Drizzle with soy sauce and serve!

ROAST CHICKEN WITH GARLIC AND HERB BUTTER:

PREP TIME: 25 MIN / COOKING TIME: 60 MIN / SERVINGS: 4 / SERVING SIZE: 1
CALORIES: 984 / NET CARBS: 0.3G / FIBRE: 0G / FAT: 82G / PROTEIN: 58G

INGREDIENTS:

- 1.5 kg // 3lb whole chicken
- 150g // 5oz homemade garlic and herb butter (see recipe)
- 2 yellow onions, cut into quarters
- Pinch of salt and pepper

METHOD:

1. Preheat the oven to 175c or 350f.

2. Place the whole chicken into a baking dish and liberally cover in the herb butter. Scatter chunks of the onion in the bottom of the dish and season liberally with salt and pepper.

3. Bake for 60 minutes, constantly basting with the melted garlic and herb butter to keep the chicken moist. Test the chicken with a meat thermometer nearing the end, it should read 75c or 165f when it's ready.

4. Serve with steamed green vegetables, or slice it for use in salads, soups or sandwiches.

MEXICAN CHILLI STUFFED PEPPERS WITH CHEESE:

PREP TIME: 10 MIN / COOKING TIME: 45 MIN / SERVINGS: 4 / SERVING SIZE: 1
CALORIES: 896 / NET CARBS: 13G / FIBRE: 5G / FAT: 70G / PROTEIN: 51G

INGREDIENTS:

- 4 green bell peppers
- 4tbsp olive oil
- 1 yellow onion, chopped finely
- 2 garlic cloves, chopped finely
- 650g // 1 ½ lb beef mince
- 2tsp chilli powder
- 2tsp cumin powder
- 200g // 7oz canned chopped tomatoes
- 225g // ½ lb grated cheese
- 225ml // 1 cup sour cream

METHOD:

1. Preheat the oven to 200c or 400f.

2. Slice the peppers in half and arrange on a baking tray.

3. Fry the onion, garlic, spices and beef mince till browned. Pour in the canned chopped tomatoes and let simmer for 15 minutes until thick.

4. Spoon the beef chilli into the halved peppers, top with grated cheese and bake in the preheated oven for 25 minutes, until the peppers are soft and the cheese is brown and bubbling.

5. Remove from the oven and serve with a generous dollop of sour cream.

SAUCES, DIPS AND CONDIMENTS

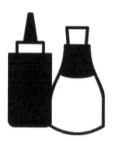

EASY KETO BECHAMEL SAUCE:

PREP TIME: 2 MIN / COOKING TIME: 15 MIN / SERVINGS: 6 CUPS / SERVING SIZE: 1 CUP
CALORIES: 351 / NET CARBS: 4G / FIBRE: 0G / FAT: 36G / PROTEIN: 4G

Recipe Note: *This creamy bechamel sauce is really simple, but absolutely delicious! It can be used in a whole array of keto friendly dishes from our special lasagne, steak sauce, salad dressing and even as a pie filling!*

INGREDIENTS:

- 425 ml // 1 ¾ cups heavy whipping cream
- 200g // 7oz cream cheese
- ¼ tsp salt
- ¼ tsp black pepper
- ¼ ground nutmeg

METHOD:

1. Add all ingredients to a large non-stick saucepan and gently bring to the boil. Keep stirring continuously or your sauce may burn!

2. Lower the heat and let your sauce simmer until the desired consistency is reached.

3. Taste your sauce and add any additional seasoning or nutmeg to suit your taste or recipe.

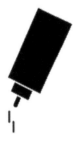

WAYNE A. COLE

LOW- CARB TOMATO SAUCE:

PREP TIME: 10 MIN / COOKING TIME: 30 MIN / SERVINGS: 16 PORTIONS / SERVING SIZE: ¼ CUP
CALORIES: 17 / NET CARBS: 1G / FIBRE: 1G / FAT: 1G / PROTEIN: 0.4G

INGREDIENTS:

- 1 tbsp olive oil
- ½ yellow onion, finely chopped
- 1 crushed garlic clove
- 2 tbsp tomato paste
- 75ml // ⅓ cup balsamic vinegar
- 1 tsp salt
- 1 bay leaf

- 1 tsp smoked paprika powder
- 1 tsp coriander seeds
- ½ tsp cloves
- ½ tsp black pepper
- 1 pinch cayenne pepper
- 400g // 14 oz. tinned tomatoes

METHOD:

1. In a deep non-stick saucepan, add the olive oil, chopped onion, garlic and tomato paste. Fry on a low heat for a few minutes until the onions are becoming soft and glossy.

2. Pour over the tinned tomatoes and vinegar, then add the bay leaves and spices. Stir continuously on a medium heat for 20 minutes.

3. Remove the bay leaf and transfer the mixture to a blender. Be careful, it will be very hot! If you're unsure about your blender, let the mixture cool slightly or it may break your appliance!

4. Wizz up until smooth and thick, taste and adjust the flavor with a little salt and pepper.

5. If your tomato sauce is too runny, you can transfer it back into the pan and continue to simmer until it has reduced enough to meet your desired consistency.

INFUSED OLIVE OIL:

PREP TIME: 5 MIN / COOKING TIME: 48 HOURS / SERVINGS: 100 / SERVING SIZE: 1TSP (5ML)
CALORIES: 40 / NET CARBS: 0G / FIBRE: 0G / FAT: 4.5G / PROTEIN: 0G

Recipe Note: Making your own infused oils is not only a great way to add flavour to your meal, but to ensure you're getting enough healthy, non-animal derived fats in your diet plan!

INGREDIENTS:

♦ 500ml olive oil

♦ Flavoring ideas - chill, garlic, black pepper, sun dried tomatoes, rosemary, thyme, lemon zest

METHOD:

1. Wash and sterilize an old glass bottle of jam jar with hot water! (Not too hot or the glass may shatter!)

2. Depending on what you use, wash, chop and tie your flavoring together well. We recommend herbs such as rosemary or thyme, or fresh chilli or garlic.

3. Carefully put your items into the glass container, and then top up with olive oil. Ensure your flavorings are fully submerged in the oil to prevent mould growing.

4. Seal and store your oils somewhere cool and dark. They'll already taste delicious after just 48 hours, but the flavour will intensify over time.

HOMEMADE ALMOND-BUTTER:

PREP TIME: 5 MIN / COOKING TIME: 20 MINUTES / SERVINGS: 12 / SERVING SIZE: 3TBSP
CALORIES: 120 / NET CARBS: 2G / FIBRE: 0G / FAT: 11G / PROTEIN: 4G

INGREDIENTS:

- 225g // 1/2 lb raw almonds (with or without their skin)
- 1tbsp coconut oil
- 1 pinch of sea salt

METHOD:

1. Preheat your oven to 150 degrees celsius (300 degrees fahrenheit).

2. Spred the almonds out evenly on a baking tray and roast in the oven for about 20 minutes, or until the nuts are golden and evenly coloured. You can turn the nuts with a spatula or shake the tray a little to ensure the almonds get toasted evenly.

3. Let the nuts cool properly. Be careful handling them straight out of the oven as they get surprisingly hot!

4. Once cool, transfer nuts to a high power blender or hand-held electric coffee bean grinder. Add the salt and coconut oil.

5. Blend properly, until the nut butter has a creamy and smooth texture. This might take some time depending on your kitchen appliance, but persevere!

Recipe Note: You can blanch your almonds to get the skin off, resulting in a much creamier smoother nut butter! To do this, simply blanch your nuts in hot water for 60 seconds, rinse with cold water and pat dry with a paper towel. You'll notice the skins will come off easily in your fingers!

You can use almost any other nut to make nut butters in this way - Macadamia, Walnut, Hazelnut etc! Check the Nutrition facts and make sure to use a low-carb nut to keep it Keto!

AVOCADO HUMMUS:

PREP TIME: 1 MIN / COOKING TIME: 5 MINUTES / SERVINGS: 6 / SERVING SIZE: ½ CUP
CALORIES: 417 / NET CARBS: 4G / FIBRE: 8G / FAT: 41G / PROTEIN: 5G

INGREDIENTS:

- 3 ripe avocados
- 125ml // ½ cup coriander (fresh)
- 125ml // ½ cup olive oil
- 35g sunflower seeds
- 60ml // ¼ cup tahini
- 1tbsp lemon juice
- 1 garlic clove
- ½ tsp ground cumin
- ½ tsp salt
- ¼ tsp black pepper

METHOD:

1. Carefully slice your avocado's lengthwise in half and twist to open. Remove the pit and scoop out the flesh with a spoon.

2. Add all of the measured ingredients to a food processor and blend for 30-60 seconds depending on the desired texture.

3. Adjust texture, consistency and taste with more seasoning, oil or lemon juice.

4. Serve with a scattering of fresh coriander leaves and a few sunflower seeds.

ALFREDO SAUCE:

PREP TIME: 1 MIN / COOKING TIME: 10 MINUTES / SERVINGS: 6 / SERVING SIZE: ¼ CUP
CALORIES: 253 / NET CARBS: 3G / FIBRE: 0G / FAT: 25G / PROTEIN: 3G

INGREDIENTS:

- 6 cloves of garlic
- 1tbsp butter
- 375mls // 12floz (1.5 cups) heavy cream
- 45g // ½ cup parmesan cheese
- Salt and pepper to taste
- Nutmeg (optional)

METHOD:

1. Mince or finely chop the garlic and sautee in the melted butter on a medium heat until fragrant (around 30 seconds).

2. Add the cream and simmer for approximately five minutes (depending on the size of your pan) until it begins to thicken and has reduced by a third.

3. Turn your heat down to low and in the parmesan cheese, whisking until smooth.

4. Stir in your seasonings to your preferred taste and then adjust thickness by either cooking for longer, or adding a touch more cream to thin it out again.

HOLLANDAISE SAUCE:

PREP TIME: 5 MIN / COOKING TIME: 5 MIN / SERVINGS: 4 / SERVING SIZE: 1
CALORIES: 174 / NET CARBS: 1G / FIBRE: 0G / FAT: 162G / PROTEIN: 2G

INGREDIENTS:
- 3 egg yolks
- 8 tbsp salted butter
- 1tbsp lemon juice
- Pinch of salt and pepper

METHOD:

1. Melt the butter slowly in a small pot on the stove. Try and only gently melt it, so it remains cloudy and does not begin to sizzle! Remove from the heat.

2. Crack eggs and separate yolks from the whites! (You can keep the whites for a high-protein omelette!)

3. Whisk the egg yolks, lemon juice and seasoning. Keep whisking vigorously until the liquid is thick and a pale yellow colour. This might take a few minutes but persevere!

4. Bring about 2 inches of water to the boil in a small saucepan. Place a pyrex or heat safe bowl over the top, ensuring the bottom of the bowl isn't touching the water. This is called a 'Bain-Marie'.

5. Pour the egg mixture into the bain-marie and whisk constantly, slowly pouring in a little melted butter at a time. Make sure the water is only gently simmering as if it's too hot your eggs will scramble!

6. After about 5 minutes of whisking and adding butter, your sauce should be thickening beautifully, and have a glossy, silky texture.

7. Remove from the heat but keep warm in a jug or bowl.

CAESAR SALAD DRESSING:

PREP TIME: 5 MIN / COOKING TIME: 5 MIN / SERVINGS: 4 / SERVING SIZE: 1
CALORIES: 156 / NET CARBS: 1G / FIBRE: 0G / FAT: 143G / PROTEIN: 1G

INGREDIENTS:
- ½ cup mayonnaise
- 1tbsp dijon mustard
- ½ lemon, juice and zest
- ½ oz grated parmesan cheese
- 2tbsp chopped anchovies
- 1 garlic clove
- Pinch of salt and pepper

METHOD:
1. Put all the ingredients in a blender and process until smooth and creamy. Keep the dressing in the fridge until you need it.

HERB BUTTER:

PREP TIME: 2 MIN / COOKING TIME: 0 MIN / SERVINGS: 4 / SERVING SIZE: 1
CALORIES: 50 / NET CARBS: 2G / FIBRE: 0G / FAT: 20G / PROTEIN: 13G

INGREDIENTS:
- 175g // 6oz salted butter
- 1 garlic clove
- ½ tsp garlic powder
- 60ml // ¼ cup chopped fresh parsley
- 1tsp fresh lemon juice
- ½ salt

METHOD:
1. Make the herb butter by mixing all ingredients together in a bowl. You may need to let the butter soften at room temperature first. Store in the fridge until you need it.

NICOISE SALAD DRESSING:

PREP TIME: 5 MIN / COOKING TIME: 0 MIN / SERVINGS: 2 / SERVING SIZE: 1
CALORIES: 32 / NET CARBS: 9G / FIBRE:0G / FAT: 10G / PROTEIN: 8G

INGREDIENTS:

- ½ tsp dijon mustard
- 2tbsp capers
- 15g // ½ anchovy
- 75ml // ⅓ cup olive oil
- 60ml // ¼ cup mayonnaise
- 1 tbsp fresh chopped parsley or chives
- ½ lemon, squeezed
- 1 garlic clove

METHOD:

1. Chop the anchovy, capers, herbs and garlic finely. Squeeze in the lemon and discard the rind.

2. Alternatively, mix all ingredients in a food processor and blend until smooth.

CREAMY MUSTARD VINAIGRETTE

PREP TIME: 5 MIN / COOKING TIME: 0 MIN / SERVINGS: 4 / SERVING SIZE: 1
CALORIES: 102 / NET CARBS: 1G / FIBRE: 0G / FAT: 31G / PROTEIN: 5G

INGREDIENTS:

- 250g // 1 ½ cups mayonnaise
- ¾ tbsp dijon mustard
- ¾ tbsp cider vinegar
- Pinch of salt and pepper

METHOD:

1. To make the dressing, mix the mayonnaise with the mustard and vinegar in a bowl and season to taste.

VERY VERSATILE CREAMY SALAD DRESSING

PREP TIME: 3 MIN / COOKING TIME: 0 MIN / SERVINGS: 3 / SERVING SIZE: 1
CALORIES: 156 / NET CARBS: 1G / FIBRE: 0G / FAT: 63G / PROTEIN: 2G

INGREDIENTS:

- 3tbsp olive oil
- 175ml // ¾ cup mayonnaise
- 2tsp lemon juice
- 1 garlic clove, finely chopped or minced
- ½ tsp salt
- ¼ tsp chilli powder

METHOD:

1. Whisk all ingredients together in a bowl and keep in the fridge until you need it.

CHIPOTLE AIOLI:

PREP TIME: 1 MIN / COOKING TIME: 0 MIN / SERVINGS: 2 / SERVING SIZE: 1
CALORIES: 96 / NET CARBS: 0G / FIBRE: 0G / FAT: 56G / PROTEIN: 1G

INGREDIENTS:

- 75ml // ⅓ cup mayonnaise
- 1tbsp smoked paprika
- 1 garlic clove, minced
- 1tsp chipotle tabasco (or other spicy sauce)

METHOD:

1. Mix together all of the ingredients in a bowl.

KETO FRIENDLY RASPBERRY JAM:

PREP TIME: 10 MIN / COOKING TIME: 0 MIN / SERVINGS: 4 / SERVING SIZE: 1
CALORIES: 30 / NET CARBS: 2G / FIBRE: 3G / FAT: 1G / PROTEIN: 1G

INGREDIENTS:

- 110g // 4oz raspberries
- 12g // 1tbsp chia seeds
- ¼ tsp vanilla essence
- 3tbsp hot water

METHOD:

1. In a bowl, pour the hot water over the chia seeds and let cool.

2. Add the vanilla essence and stir. Tip in the fresh raspberries and mash or blend with a hand blender, depending on how smooth you like your jam to be.

3. Once cooled down, transfer to a glass jar and put in the fridge, within 4 hours your jam should have set and will be ready to use.

EGGPLANT DIP:

PREP TIME: 5 MIN / COOKING TIME: 30 MIN / SERVINGS: 6 / SERVING SIZE: 1
CALORIES: 123 / NET CARBS: 3G / FIBRE: 11G / FAT: 11G / PROTEIN: 2G

INGREDIENTS:

- 600g // 20oz eggplant
- ½ tsp cumin powder
- 60ml // ¼ cup olive oil
- 1tbsp lemon juice
- 2tbsp sesame seeds
- Pinch of salt and pepper

METHOD:

1. Char the eggplant directly over a gas hob flame. The skin will bubble and turn black when it's ready.

2. Run the charred eggplants under a cold tap to cool down. Slice lengthways and use a spoon to scoop out the soft insides. Discard the blackened skin.

3. Add to a bowl the lemon juice, cumin, olive oil, sesame seeds and seasoning. Mash with a fork until the dip is thick and creamy.

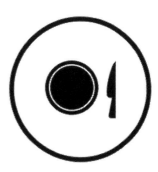

DESSERTS

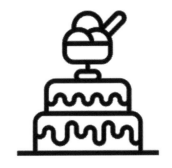

DARK CHOCOLATE CUPS:

PREP TIME: 10 MIN / COOKING TIME: 60 MIN / SERVINGS: 20 / SERVING SIZE: 1
CALORIES: 79 / NET CARBS: 4G / FIBRE: 1G / FAT: 6G / PROTEIN: 1G

INGREDIENTS:
- 100g // 3 ½ oz dark chocolate
- 10 whole hazelnuts
- 2tbsp toasted coconut flakes
- 1tbsp pumpkin seeds
- Pinch of sea salt

METHOD:
1. Melt the chocolate gradually in a bowl over a pan of hot water.
2. Place 10 small cupcake liners out on a baking tray, fill each with 2 tablespoons of the melted dark chocolate.
3. Decorate with the nuts, seeds and a pinch of sea salt. Place in the fridge to chill and serve once set!

FRESH BERRIES WITH WHIPPED CREAM:

PREP TIME: 15 MIN / COOKING TIME: 0 MIN / SERVINGS: 2 / SERVING SIZE: 1
CALORIES: 307 / NET CARBS: 6G / FIBRE: 5G / FAT: 29G / PROTEIN: 3G

INGREDIENTS:
- 150g // 5oz fresh berries, such as raspberries, strawberries or blueberries
- 150ml // ⅔ cup double cream
- ¼ tsp vanilla essence
- Bunch of fresh mint as a garnish

METHOD:
1. Whip the cream and vanilla essence together with an electric mixer, till it forms stiff peaks.
2. Divide cream between bowls and arrange the fresh berries on top. Garnish with a few sprigs of fresh mint.

CHOCOLATE MACADAMIA BONBONS:

PREP TIME: 10 MIN / COOKING TIME: 30 MIN / SERVINGS: 4 / SERVING SIZE: 1
CALORIES: 167 / NET CARBS: 2G / FIBRE: 2G / FAT: 16G / PROTEIN: 2G

INGREDIENTS:

- 40g // 1 ⅓ oz dark chocolate
- 1tbsp butter
- 40g // 1 ½ oz macadamia nuts
- Pinch of sea salt

METHOD:

1. Melt the butter, sea salt and chocolate together, in a bowl over a pan of hot water.

2. Using a silicone truffle or ice cube tray, place 1 teaspoon of the melted chocolate mixture at the bottom. Carefully place 1 macadamia nut on top of each.

3. Cover with the remaining chocolate and put in the fridge to set for 1 hour. The chocolate bonbon's should pop out of the moulds easily once set.

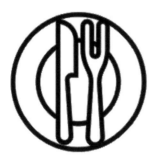

SPICED CHAI TRUFFLE BALLS:

PREP TIME: 10 MIN / COOKING TIME: 35 MIN / SERVINGS: 10 / SERVING SIZE: 1
CALORIES: 91 / NET CARBS: 1G / FIBRE: 1G / FAT: 10G / PROTEIN: 0.4G

INGREDIENTS:

- 75g // 3oz butter
- 50g // ½ cup shredded coconut
- 1tsp ground cinnamon
- 1tsp ground cardamom
- ½ tsp vanilla essence

METHOD:

1. Toast the coconut in a dry frying pan until light brown in colour. Remove from the heat and let cool.

2. Mix half the coconut with the butter, vanilla essence, cinnamon and cardamom and stir until fully blended. Let cool in the fridge until it's stiffer and easier to handle.

3. Roll tablespoon amounts of the mixture between the palms of your hands. Once firm little balls, roll in the leftover toasted coconut and put on a plate. Refrigerate and serve!

LEMON ICE CREAM:

PREP TIME: 30 MIN / COOKING TIME: 60 MIN / SERVINGS: 6 / SERVING SIZE: 1
CALORIES: 269 / NET CARBS: 3G / FIBRE: 0G / FAT: 27G / PROTEIN: 5G

INGREDIENTS:

- 1 lemon
- 3 eggs
- 50g // ⅓ cup erythritol sweetener
- 425ml // 1 ¾ cup double cream

METHOD:

1. Zest and juice the lemon and set aside.

2. Seperate the eggs into different bowls. Whisk the egg whites until it forms stiff peaks. Beat the yolks with the erythritol sweetener, lemon zest and lemon juice until light in colour and creamy.

3. Whisk the double cream until its forming stiff peaks, then fold in both the egg whites and the egg yolk mixture carefully.

4. Transfer to an ice cream maker, or a tupperware container and freeze. If freezing, keep stirring the ice cream every 30 minutes, until the ice cream reaches its desired consistency.

VANILLA BEAN PANNA COTTA:

PREP TIME: 10 MIN / COOKING TIME: 3 HOURS / SERVINGS: 4 / SERVING SIZE: 1
CALORIES: 422 / NET CARBS: 4G / FIBRE: 0G / FAT: 43G / PROTEIN: 4G

INGREDIENTS:

- 2tsp powdered gelatine dissolved in water
- 2 cups double cream
- 1tsp vanilla bean paste
- 1tsp erythritol sweetener

METHOD:

1. Mix double cream, vanilla and sweetener to a saucepan and bring to the boil. Once bubbling reduce the heat and let it simmer for 3-5 minutes, or until the cream begins to thicken.

2. Remove the cream from the heat and gradually stir in the gelatine liquid until it's all dissolved and fully incorporated.

3. Pour the panna cotta mixture into glasses or ramekins and chill for 3 hours. Serve with fresh berries and a few sprigs of mint.

BLUEBERRY ICE CREAM:

PREP TIME: 30 MIN / COOKING TIME: 60 MIN / SERVINGS: 6 / SERVING SIZE: 1
CALORIES: 269 / NET CARBS: 3G / FIBRE: 0G / FAT: 27G / PROTEIN: 5G

INGREDIENTS:

- 175g // 6oz frozen blueberries
- ½ tsp cinnamon
- 3 eggs
- 50g // ⅓ cup erythritol sweetener
- 425ml // 1 ¾ cup double cream

METHOD:

1. Microwave the frozen blueberries and cinnamon for 3 minutes, until they're thawed out and have become a jammy consistency.

2. Seperate the eggs into different bowls. Whisk the egg whites until they form stiff peaks. Beat the yolks with the erythritol sweetener and blueberry jam until light in colour and creamy.

3. Whisk the double cream until its forming stiff peaks, then fold in both the egg whites and the egg yolk mixture carefully.

4. Transfer to an ice cream maker, or a tupperware container and freeze. If freezing, keep stirring the ice cream every 30 minutes until the ice cream reaches its desired consistency.

CINNAMON APPLE TRIFLE:

PREP TIME: 20 MIN / COOKING TIME: 20 MIN / SERVINGS: 6 / SERVING SIZE: 1
CALORIES: 476 / NET CARBS: 12G / FIBRE: 2G / FAT: 47G / PROTEIN: 4G

INGREDIENTS:

- 5tbsp butter
- 3 apples
- 1tbsp ground cinnamon
- 600ml // double cream
- ½ tsp vanilla essence
- 1 egg yolk

METHOD:

1. Place the butter, vanilla and half the double cream in a pan and bring to the boil, let simmer for 5 minutes until the cream has thickened. Remove from the heat and once cool, beat in the egg yolk. Transfer the creamy custard to the fridge and let chill.

2. Core and slice the apples thinly and sprinkle with cinnamon. Fry the apple slices in butter until they are soft and juicy.

3. Whip the remaining double cream till it forms stiff peaks.

4. Assemble the trifle with layers of custard, apple and cream. Dust with a little cinnamon and serve.

AVOCADO CHOCOLATE TRUFFLES:

PREP TIME: 35 MIN / COOKING TIME: 20 MIN / SERVINGS: 20 / SERVING SIZE: 1
CALORIES: 65 / NET CARBS: 3G / FIBRE: 2G / FAT: 5G / PROTEIN: 1G

INGREDIENTS:

- 1 avocado
- ½ tsp vanilla essence
- ½ lime, zested
- 1 pinch of sea salt
- 150g // 5oz 80% cocoa dark chocolate
- 1tbsp coconut oil
- 5g // 1tbsp cocoa powder

METHOD:

1. Mash the avocado with the vanilla essence until completely smooth and lump free (or you can use a food processor). Stir in the lime zest and sea salt.

2. Melt the coconut oil and dark chocolate in a bowl over a pan of boiling water.

3. Mix together the melted chocolate and avocado mixture and chill in the fridge for 30 minutes, or until the mixture has stiffened up enough to be handled.

4. Roll teaspoon sized truffle balls between the palms of your hands, coat in cocoa powder and serve!

SUMMER BERRY CRUMBLE POTS:

PREP TIME: 5 MIN / COOKING TIME: 15 MIN / SERVINGS: 4 / SERVING SIZE: 1
CALORIES: 315 / NET CARBS: 5G / FIBRE: 8G / FAT: 27G / PROTEIN: 7G

INGREDIENTS:

- 275 // 10oz fresh berries, such as blueberries, strawberries and raspberries
- 2tbsp lime juice
- 1tsp cinnamon
- 250g // 1 cup homemade nutty granola (see recipe)

METHOD:

1. Stew the berries, lime juice and cinnamon in a small saucepan over a low heat for 15 minutes, until they have broken down into a jammy consistency. Set aside to cool

2. Serve spoonfuls of the cooled berry's in jars, with our homemade nutty granola on top. Can be served hot or cold and will be delicious served with a generous dollop of whipped double cream!

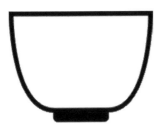

CHOCOLATE FUDGE BARS:

PREP TIME: 5 MIN / COOKING TIME: 30 MIN / SERVINGS: 24 / SERVING SIZE: 1
CALORIES: 118 / NET CARBS: 2G / FIBRE: 0G / FAT: 12G / PROTEIN: 1G

INGREDIENTS:

- 480ml // 2 cups double cream
- 1tsp vanilla essence
- 90g // 3oz butter
- 90g // 3oz dark chocolate

METHOD:

1. Pour double cream and vanilla essence into a saucepan and bring to the boil. Simmer for about 20 minutes, until the cream is thickening and has halved in volume.

2. Lower the heat and add the butter, stirring until everything has melted. Remove from the heat and add the chopped dark chocolate. Keep stirring until the chocolate has melted. At this stage you can add any other flavorings you like, such as peppermint extract, orange zest or chopped nuts.

3. Pour the mixture into a lined baking dish and chill for 30 minutes. Chop into squares and serve cold.

FRUITY FROZEN YOGHURT:

PREP TIME: 10 MIN / COOKING TIME: 2 HOURS / SERVINGS: 12 / SERVING SIZE: 1
CALORIES: 72 / NET CARBS: 5G / FIBRE: 1G / FAT: 5G / PROTEIN: 2G

INGREDIENTS:
- 225g // 8oz frozen mango, chopped into small pieces
- 225g // 8oz frozen strawberries, chopped into small pieces
- 225ml // 1 cup greek yoghurt
- 125ml // ½ double cream
- 1tsp vanilla essence

METHOD:
1. Combine all ingredients in a food processor and blend for 30 seconds.
2. Pour into a tupperware container and freeze. Once frozen, scoop out and blend again till creamy. Serve with chopped up fresh fruit!

GRIDDLED HOT PEACHES WITH CREAM:

PREP TIME: 15 MIN / COOKING TIME: 5 MIN / SERVINGS: 4 / SERVING SIZE: 1
CALORIES: 298 / NET CARBS: 11G / FIBRE: 2G / FAT: 27G / PROTEIN: 3G

INGREDIENTS:
- 3 ripe peaches
- 1tsp ground cinnamon
- 2tbsp coconut oil
- 225ml // 1 cup double cream
- Sprigs of mint to garnish

METHOD:
1. Whip the cream and set aside.
2. Cut the peaches in half and remove the stones. Slice into chunky segments. Mix in a bowl with the coconut oil and cinnamon and cover liberally.
3. Grill the peaches on a bbq, or with a griddle pan on the stove until lightly cooked and browning on the outside. Serve warm with cream and a few mint leaves.

NUTTY GRANOLA BARS WITH DARK CHOCOLATE:

PREP TIME: 10 MIN / COOKING TIME: 20 MIN / SERVINGS: 20 / SERVING SIZE: 1
CALORIES: 476 / NET CARBS: 12G / FIBRE: 2G / FAT: 47G / PROTEIN: 4G

INGREDIENTS:

- 110g // 4oz pecan nuts, hazelnuts or almonds (or a mixture of all three)
- 35g // 1 ¼ oz shredded coconut
- 75g // ½ cup sunflower seeds
- 15g // 2tbsp pumpkin seeds
- 20g // 2tbsp sesame seeds

- 75g // ⅖ cup flax seeds
- ½ turmeric
- ½ cinnamon powder
- 1tsp vanilla essence
- 30g // ¼ cup almond flour
- 8 tbsp coconut oil
- 75g // 3oz dark chocolate

METHOD:

1. First, preheat the oven to 150c, or 65f.

2. Crush and chop the nuts coarsely with a sharp knife.

3. Mix all of the ingredients together in a large bowl. You may need to melt the coconut oil slightly if it has solidified. Simply put it in the microwave for 30 seconds to melt!

4. Spoon mixture out onto a greaseproof paper lined baking tray and spread out evenly. Bake in the oven for about 30 minutes, or until the nutty mixture is golden and crunchy. Remove from the oven.

5. Drizzle with melted dark chocolate and place in the fridge to cool. Cut into rough squares and serve.

CHOCOLATE AND RASPBERRY MOUSSE:

PREP TIME: 5 MIN / COOKING TIME: 1 HOUR / SERVINGS: 6 / SERVING SIZE: 1
CALORIES: 270 / NET CARBS: 6G / FIBRE: 2G / FAT: 25G / PROTEIN: 3G

INGREDIENTS:

- 300ml // 1 ¼ cup double cream
- ½ tsp vanilla essence
- 2 egg yolks
- 1 pinch of sea salt
- 75g // 3oz dark 80% cocoa chocolate

METHOD:

1. Melt the chocolate with the vanilla and sea salt in a bowl over a pan of hot water.

2. Whisk the cream till it forms stiff peaks. In a separate bowl, whisk the egg yolk until it's pale and creamy.

3. Slowly fold the melted chocolate and whisked egg yolk into the cream. Divide into glasses and chill in the fridge for 1 hour. Serve with fresh raspberries on the top.

SNACKS

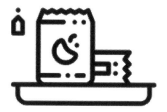

CHEESE CRISPS:

PREP TIME: 5 MIN / COOKING TIME: 5 MIN / SERVINGS: 4 / SERVING SIZE: 1
CALORIES: 156 / NET CARBS: 1G / FIBRE: 0G / FAT: 143G / PROTEIN: 1G

INGREDIENTS:
- 125g // 4 ½ oz cheddar cheese
- ½ tsp paprika powder

METHOD:
1. To make the cheese crisps, place spoonfuls of grated cheese on a greaseproof paper lined baking tray. Sprinkle the little piles of cheese with paprika.

2. Grill in the oven on a high temperature for 5-6 minutes, until the cheese has melted and begun to bubble. Remove from the oven and let cool fully before removing the chips from the tray.

HALLOUMI AND BACON BITES:

PREP TIME: 10 MIN / COOKING TIME: 10 MIN / SERVINGS: 2 / SERVING SIZE: 1
CALORIES: 705 / NET CARBS: 4G / FIBRE: 0G / FAT: 61G / PROTEIN: 34G

INGREDIENTS:
- 225g // 8oz halloumi cheese
- 175g // 6oz streaky bacon

METHOD:
1. Cut cheese into chip size lengths and wrap with bacon.

2. Fry or bake in the oven at 200c, 400f, until golden brown and crunchy.

GARLIC BREAD

PREP TIME: 5 MIN / COOKING TIME: 5 MIN / SERVINGS: 8 / SERVING SIZE: 1
CALORIES: 94 / NET CARBS: 1G / FIBRE: 2G / FAT: 9G / PROTEIN: 2G

INGREDIENTS:

- 8 slices of keto friendly bread - cloud bread/mug bread/no-nuts bread etc
- 4tbsp garlic and herb butter (see recipe)

METHOD:

1. Spread the bread slices with garlic and herb butter.
2. Grill on a high heat for 5 minutes, until the butter is bubbling and the bread has turned golden brown.

VEGETABLE STICKS WITH AVOCADO HUMMUS:

PREP TIME: 5 MIN / COOKING TIME: 0 / SERVINGS: 4 / SERVING SIZE: 1
CALORIES: 696 / NET CARBS: 8G / FIBRE: 2G / FAT: 68G / PROTEIN: 12G

INGREDIENTS:

- 1 small carrot
- 1 green pepper
- 3 celery sticks
- 1 small cucumber
- 500ml // 2 cups avocado hummus (see recipe)

METHOD:

1. Chop vegetables lengthways into neat little sticks.
2. Serve with a bowl of avocado hummus, or your choice of keto-friendly dressing or sauce for dipping.

SPICY ROAST NUTS

PREP TIME: 5 MIN / COOKING TIME: 10 MIN / SERVINGS: 6 / SERVING SIZE: 1
CALORIES: 285 / NET CARBS: 2G / FIBRE: 4G / FAT: 30G / PROTEIN: 4G

INGREDIENTS:

- 225g // 8oz nuts - almonds, walnuts, macadamia's etc
- 1tsp salt
- 1tbsp olive oil
- 1tsp chilli powder
- 1tsp cumin

METHOD:

1. Mix nuts with spices, seasoning and olive oil.
2. Heat in a frying pan until toasted and brown on the outside.
3. Let cool and serve as a snack.

HOMEMADE PORK SCRATCHINGS:

PREP TIME: 30 MIN / COOKING TIME: 15 MIN / SERVINGS: 4 / SERVING SIZE: 1
CALORIES: 427 / NET CARBS: 0G / FIBRE: 0G / FAT: 31G / PROTEIN: 35G

INGREDIENTS:

- 225g // 1 ½ lb pork skin
- 1tsp salt
- 475 // 2 cups oil or lard for frying

METHOD:

1. Chop the pork skin into bite sized strips. Preheat the oil or lard in a saucepan until very hot.
2. Deep fry the pork skin till it bubbles and turns golden. Remove from the oil, drain and let cool.
3. Sprinkle with sea salt and serve.

SPICY COURGETTE CRISPS:

PREP TIME: 5 MIN / COOKING TIME: 20 MINS / SERVINGS: 4 / SERVING SIZE: 1
CALORIES: 145 / NET CARBS: 2G / FIBRE: 1G / FAT: 14G / PROTEIN: 1G

INGREDIENTS:

- 1 large courgette
- Pinch of salt
- 1tsp paprika
- 1tsp chilli powder
- 350ml // 1 ½ cups olive oil

METHOD:

1. Slice the courgette into thin rounds with a sharp knife or mandolin.
2. Season with salt and spices.
3. Transfer to a baking tray, drizzle with olive oil and bake in the oven at 200c, 400f for 20 minutes, or until golden and crunchy.

MUG BREAD CRACKER THINS WITH DIP:

PREP TIME: 3 MIN / COOKING TIME: 3 MIN / SERVINGS: 2 / SERVING SIZE: 1
CALORIES:294 / NET CARBS: 3G / FIBRE: 4G / FAT: 27G / PROTEIN:9G

INGREDIENTS:

- 1 mug bread loaf (see recipe)
- 1tbsp olive oil
- Assortment of dips - Avocado hummus, chipotle aioli or caesar salad dressing

METHOD:

1. Slice the mug bread into 6 thin slices.
2. Brush with oil and grill on a baking tray for 5 minutes, until the bread is crunchy and golden.
3. Serve with your favorite dips as a quick and easy snack!

KALE CHIPS:

PREP TIME:10 MIN / COOKING TIME: 15 MINS / SERVINGS: 4 / SERVING SIZE: 1
CALORIES: 58 / NET CARBS: 3G / FIBRE: 2G / FAT: 4G / PROTEIN: 2G

INGREDIENTS:
- 225g // 1/2lb kale
- 1 tbsp olive oil
- ½ tsp lemon juice
- Pinch of salt and pepper

METHOD:

1. Chop the kale leaves into chunky strips and lay on a baking tray.

2. Drizzle with oil, lemon juice and seasoning and bake in a hot oven for 15 minutes, until crispy and dark green.

SEEDED PARMESAN CHIPS:

PREP TIME: 5 MIN / COOKING TIME: 0 MINS / SERVINGS: 2 / SERVING SIZE: 1
CALORIES: 281 / NET CARBS: 2G / FIBRE: 6G / FAT: 20G / PROTEIN: 19G

INGREDIENTS:
- 75g parmesan cheese, grated
- 1 tbsp chia seeds
- 1 tbsp flax seeds
- 1 ½ tbsp pumpkin seeds

METHOD:

1. To make the parmesan crisps, place spoonfuls of the grated cheese on a greaseproof paper lined baking tray. Sprinkle the little piles of cheese with the mixed seeds.

2. Grill in the oven on a high temperature for 5-6 minutes, until the cheese has melted and begun to bubble. Remove from the oven and let cool fully before removing the chips from the tray.

GRILLED CHEESE SANDWICH

PREP TIME: 5 MIN / COOKING TIME: 5 MIN / SERVINGS: 2 / SERVING SIZE: 1
CALORIES: 800 / NET CARBS: 7G / FIBRE: 3G / FAT: 75G / PROTEIN: 22G

INGREDIENTS:

- 150g // 5oz cheddar cheese
- 1tbsp mayonnaise
- 4 slices of no-nuts keto bread (see recipe)
- 1tbsp butter.

METHOD:

1. Spread mayonnaise on each side of the no-nuts keto bread, grate the cheese and assemble your sandwich.

2. Spread butter on the outsides of the bread and fry in a griddle pan for 5 minutes until the bread is toasted and the cheese is melted and bubbling.

3. You can also try spreading mayonnaise on the outside of the bread instead of butter - also very delicious!

CHIA SEED PUDDING WITH FRESH BERRIES:

PREP TIME: 2 MIN / COOKING TIME: OVERNIGHT / SERVINGS: 1 / SERVING SIZE: 1
CALORIES: 568 / NET CARBS: 8G / FIBRE: 8G / FAT: 56G / PROTEIN: 9G

INGREDIENTS:

- 225ml // 1 cup of chia seed pudding (see recipe)
- Fresh berries
- Almond butter or our keto-friendly raspberry jam to serve

METHOD:

1. Spoon out leftover chia seed pudding into a bowl and top with fresh berries, such as strawberries, raspberries and blueberries.

2. Serve with your favorite keto-friendly sweet sauce!

NO-NUTS TOAST WITH BUTTER:

PREP TIME: 15 MIN / COOKING TIME: 35 MIN / SERVINGS: 5 / SERVING SIZE: 2 SLICES
CALORIES: 105 / NET CARBS: 1G / FIBRE: 3G / FAT: 8G / PROTEIN: 6G

INGREDIENTS:
- 5 slices of no-nuts keto bread
- 5tsp salted butter

METHOD:
1. Toast slices of bread in a toaster or frying pan.
2. Spread with butter and enjoy!
3. You can also use up any leftover dips you have in your fridge to dunk the toast in.

BOILED EGGS WITH MAYONNAISE:

PREP TIME: 2 MIN / COOKING TIME: 10 MIN / SERVINGS: 2 / SERVING SIZE: 1
CALORIES: 316 / NET CARBS: 1G / FIBRE: 1G / FAT: 29G / PROTEIN:11G

INGREDIENTS:
- 8 eggs
- 8tbsp mayonnaise
- Pinch of salt and pepper

METHOD:
1. Fill a deep cooking pot with water and bring to the boil.
2. Once at a rolling boil, turn down the temperature and carefully add your eggs with a spoon, one at a time.
3. Boil the eggs for 5 minutes for soft boiled or 8 minutes for hard boiled.
4. Remove the eggs from the water with a slotted spoon and set to one side to cool slightly. Peel and and mash together with the mayonnaise.
5. If you're more hungry then serve with no-nuts toast with butter, or any keto-friendly bread.

SALAD WRAP BITES:

PREP TIME: 5 MIN / COOKING TIME: 0 MIN / SERVINGS: 2 / SERVING SIZE: 1
CALORIES: 383 / NET CARBS: 5G / FIBRE: 9G / FAT: 34G / PROTEIN:10G

INGREDIENTS:

- 50g // 2oz lettuce leaves - such as iceberg or romaine
- 15g // ½ oz mayonnaise
- 30g // 1oz grated cheese
- ½ avocado, sliced
- 6 cherry tomatoes, sliced.

METHOD:

1. Spread a little mayonnaise on each lettuce leaf.

2. Top with cheese, avocado and cherry tomatoes.

3. Wrap and enjoy!

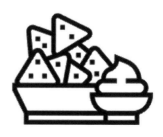

DISCLAIMER

This book contains opinions and ideas of the author and is meant to teach the reader informative and helpful knowledge while due care should be taken by the user in the application of the information provided. The instructions and strategies are possibly not right for every reader and there is no guarantee that they work for everyone. Using this book and implementing the information/recipes therein contained is explicitly your own responsibility and risk. This work with all its contents, does not guarantee correctness, completion, quality or correctness of the provided information. Misinformation or misprints cannot be completely eliminated.

Printed in Great Britain
by Amazon

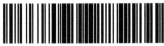

65713785R00066